OM YOGA

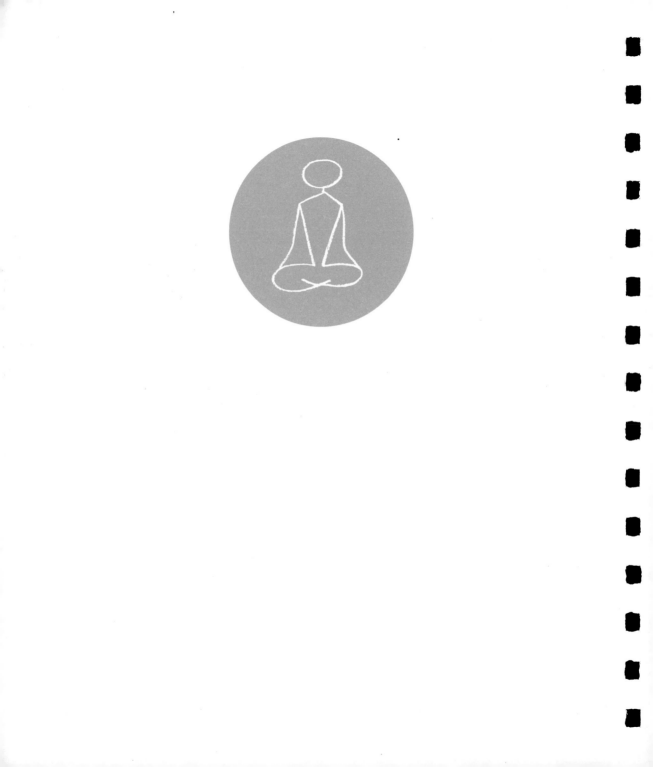

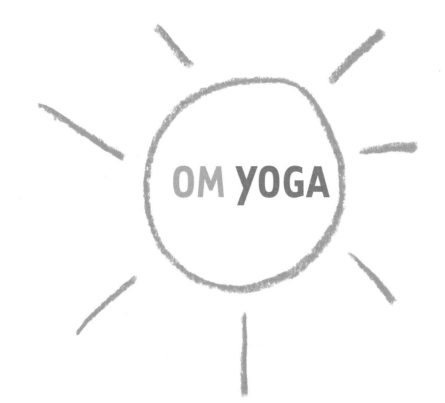

OM YOGA

A Guide to Daily Practice

WRITTEN AND ILLUSTRATED BY CYNDI LEE

CHRONICLE BOOKS
SAN FRANCISCO

Library of Congress Cataloging-in-Publication Data available.

ISBN 0-8118-3513-8

Manufactured in China.

Distributed in Canada by Raincoast Books
9050 Shaughnessy Street
Vancouver, British Columbia V6P 6E5

10 9 8 7 6

Chronicle Books LLC
85 Second Street
San Francisco, California 94105

www.chroniclebooks.com

Design by Laurie Dolphin Design

Dedication:

To my parents,
Allan and Mildred Lee
(who can both still touch their toes!)

Thank you for teaching me the two most important daily practices:
helping others and having fun.

Acknowledgments:

Thanks to the students and teachers at OM yoga center, who inspire me every day, and to OM administrative staff, especially Heather Larson Shaw and Seiko Morningstar, who cheerfully kept the studio on track while I was buried in huge piles of drawing paper. Muchas gracias to our editor, Sarah Malarkey, who is as flexible as any true yogi. Much appreciation to the Omega Institute Hermitage Program and Alison Granucci for giving me a cabin in the woods from May 13–23, 2001. As always, a big thank you to my husband, David, who never acts like he is sick of hearing about yoga. Finally, tons of appreciation to my partner, Laurie Dolphin, whose outrageousness, blind faith, and encouragement form a delicious combo platter of riches that she makes a practice of sharing daily.

Not all exercises are suitable for everyone. Your physical condition and health are important factors in determining which yoga exercises, positions, and advice may be appropriate. This or any other exercise program may result in injury. The packager, author, and publisher of this book disclaim any liability from any injury that may result from the use, proper or improper, of any exercise or advice contained in this book. Please consult your professional health care provider for information and advice on the suitability of your exercise program.

Contents

Daily Yoga Practice

Yoga invites us to harmonize our body, breath, and mind as a way to experience wakefulness and compassion in our daily lives. The path of hatha yoga involves physical exercises that enhance our cardiovascular system, strengthen our muscles, improve our digestive activity, and cleanse our entire body. It also includes breathing exercises that soothe our nervous system and meditation that develops mental clarity. The combination of these three aspects results in a sense of well-being, confidence, openheartedness, and patience.

So when we practice yoga, what we are really practicing is how to live a richer, more vivid, more connected life. Even though yoga is primarily a physical activity, the reason it enhances our entire life and even the lives of those around us is because of the mindfulness with which we approach our yoga program.

Most of us are task oriented and understand how to begin and complete a job. But yoga is never finished. It is always about the process, not the product. Each day is a fresh start. Yoga teaches us how to pay attention to our changing experiences with curiosity rather than judgment or expectation. This approach generates feelings of warmth and appreciation and a sense that life is manageable.

We're not practicing so we can be better people—more fit, happier—although those are common side effects of yoga. We're not trying to advance or to improve, to complete more missions, to gain more recognition, to attract more attention. We're simply practicing how to look at ourselves and our world with wide-open eyes and a wide-open heart. The healthy, insightful, and tender relationship with ourselves that arises from this daily practice will, in turn, nourish our relationships with others.

So we do our yoga practice every day because every day is different. What we felt yesterday will have shifted today, and when we learn to pay attention we will discover these physical shifts, openings, discomforts, releases. We will also begin to recognize our emotional and mental patterns—our habits, our cravings, our fears—and to watch how they change in the same way that we watch our tight hips begin to release or our weak abdominals grow strong.

Yoga practice is made up of a series of postures called *asanas*. *Asana* is sometimes translated as "to sit with." Let your daily yoga practice be a time to sit with yourself, to let go of your agenda, to make your own acquaintance.

You will find that over time your yoga practice will not only give you a stronger body, deeper breathing, and a more stabilized and spacious mind, but it will also awaken your senses and open your heart. Anyone can experience this. All that is required is a touch of bravery, a dose of discipline, a lot of curiosity, and of course, daily practice.

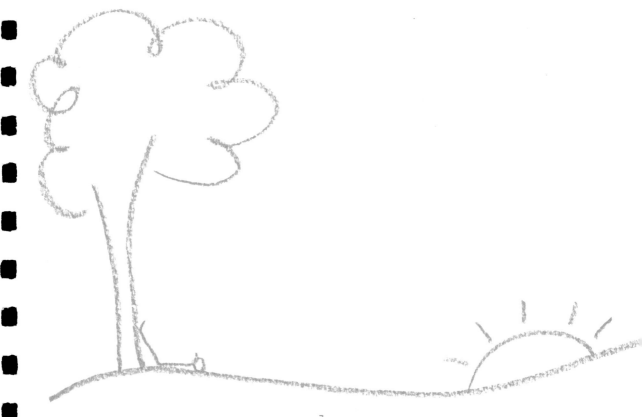

How to Use This Book

To create a daily yoga practice, simply follow the chapters in order. Every day you will first take your seat on a cushion and then begin your breathing awareness exercises. You can chant Om silently or out loud. Then you will do the daily warm-up sequence. Next you will turn the page for whatever day it is and follow that program.

Since each day is different I have designed a daily program to suit each day of the week. Although each day has a specific focus, each program is a complete practice that includes forward bending, backward bending, standing poses, twists, inversions, and side bends in a *vinyasa* format. (*Vinyasa* is a flowing style of yoga in which poses are joined by transitional movements and coordinated with rhythmic breathing patterns.)

The sequence of the week's yoga programs follows the traditional method for learning yoga:

* **Sun salute** generates energy and creates heat in the body.
* **Standing poses** create strength and develop correct posture.
* **Balancing poses** teach harmony of effort and release, inner and outer awareness.
* **Seated poses** are calming to the mind and rejuvenating to the organs.
* **Back bends** encourage us to be brave and openhearted.
* **Inversions** rejuvenate the entire body/mind system.
* **Restorative poses** create a sense of relaxed awareness and teach us how to receive.

Each day's program is laid out in one spread to help you see the whole sequence at once. In the following pages, each individual pose is detailed with instructional arrows showing how to breathe, where to put your weight, how to use your muscles and bones, and so on.

After you have completed the sequence for a given day, wind down your yoga session with the daily relaxation, chant Om three times, and dedicate your practice.

Follow this with a sitting meditation. If you have time, you can also do a walking meditation or incorporate one into your day's activities. Hopefully all your practice insights and experiences will begin to seep into the activities and awareness of your daily life.

As your body becomes stronger, your breath deeper, and your mind more stable, you will be able to lengthen your practice. At that point you will still begin with the daily warm-up and finish with the daily relaxation, but you can add more than one day's sequence in the middle section. Refer to the recipes section to learn how to mix and match the days to create practice sessions of varying lengths or intentions—invigorating or relaxing. Your daily practice will eventually develop in length anywhere from fifteen minutes to one hour.

Good luck!

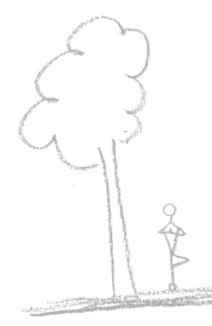

How to Sit

Begin by sitting on the floor in a comfortable cross-legged position. If the word *comfortable* and sitting on the floor don't go together for you, try placing several cushions under your sitting bones. If your cushion is square or rectangular, sit on the corner so that just your sitting bones are on the cushion, but not your thighs, allowing your knees to be at about 110 degrees lower than your hips. Lift your spine up, but keep your chest and stomach soft.

Place your palms on your thighs—this is called the mudra of calm abiding. Feel the weight of your thigh bones, calves, and feet dropping down into the earth, giving you a sense of grounding and support. Lightly press your palms down with just the weight of a nickel and feel the opposite action of lifting occur, giving a sense of buoyancy to your heart.

Whenever you notice that you've slouched, simply reorganize your sitting posture. In your mind's eye climb the ladder of your spine all the way to the very top, right between your ears. Bobble your head around, finding a delicate balance on your neck. Relax your jaw and the space between your eyes.

Rest your mind.

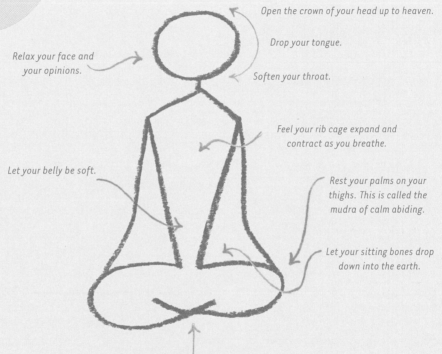

You might not find it easy to sit like this at first, but as you begin to rest your mind, you may begin to experience a sense of ease.

Open the crown of your head up to heaven.

Drop your tongue.

Soften your throat.

Relax your face and your opinions.

Feel your rib cage expand and contract as you breathe.

Let your belly be soft.

Rest your palms on your thighs. This is called the mudra of calm abiding.

Let your sitting bones drop down into the earth.

Cross your legs in a way that is comfortable for you. Try sitting on a cushion.

Easy-Pose

How to Breathe

Sitting in a comfortable cross-legged position, begin to observe your breath. Notice the ever-present tidal quality of the breath, in and out, in and out. This constant movement is our basic way of connecting with one another, because we are all breathing in and out from the same source of air. In this way breathing is an experience of both giving and receiving.

Now begin to deepen your breathing very slowly, breath by breath. Make the next inhalation slightly deeper than the one before and the next exhalation slightly longer than the one before. Make sure you are breathing both in and out through the nose, not the mouth. Keep your lips softly touching, with your teeth separated and your jaw loose.

As you inhale, feel your body expanding. Feel your belly, chest, ribs, and back filling up and extending out to the front, back, and sides. As you exhale, feel your body softening back in toward your center.

Try to make your in-breath and your out-breath equal in length.

Let your mind ride on your breath.

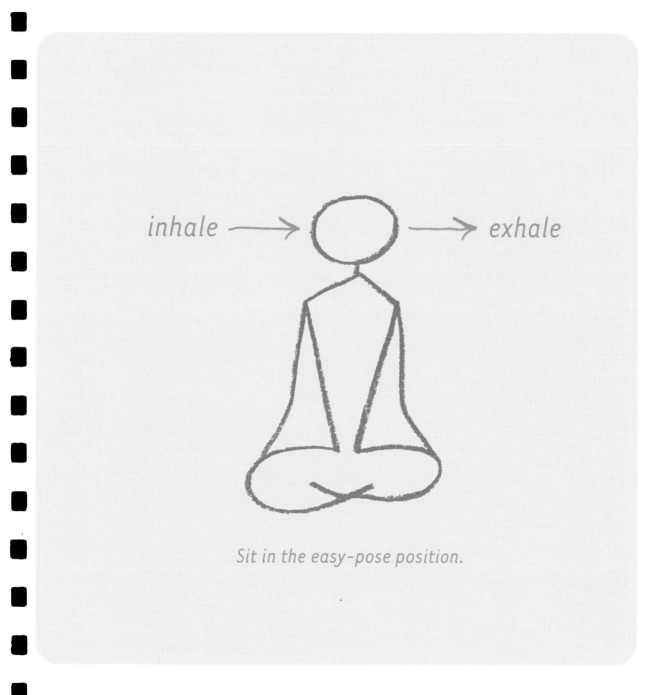

inhale → → *exhale*

Sit in the easy-pose position.

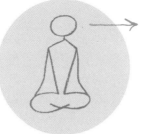

Say "Oooommmmmm" three times.

What Is Om?

Om is a mantra that we chant three times at the beginning and end of every Om yoga class. It is said to be the sound of the universe breathing. It is the sound of the waves on the shore, the wind blowing through the trees, the inside of a shell, a bird's wings. It is the sound of the ebb and flow of the ocean, the change of seasons, the movement from day to night.

Om has no origin. The entire universe expands and contracts constantly, and this pulsation creates a hum that, for centuries, people have been vocalizing as Om. So when we chant Om we remind ourselves of how we are connected to one another and to all that is.

Take a deep breath in, and as you exhale make the sound "OOOOOOOOOOOOOMMMMM-MMMMMMM."

Let your mind flow out on your breath and mix with space as you rest in the silence after Om.

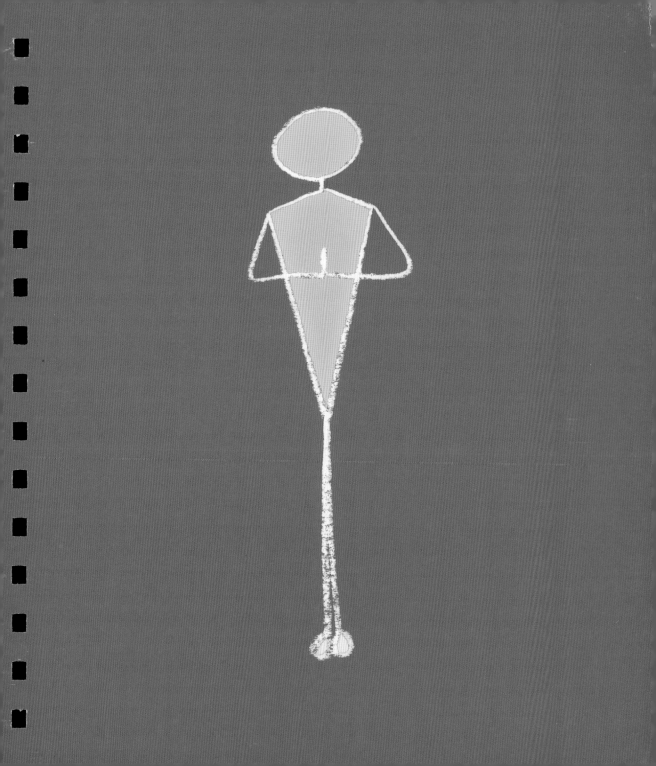

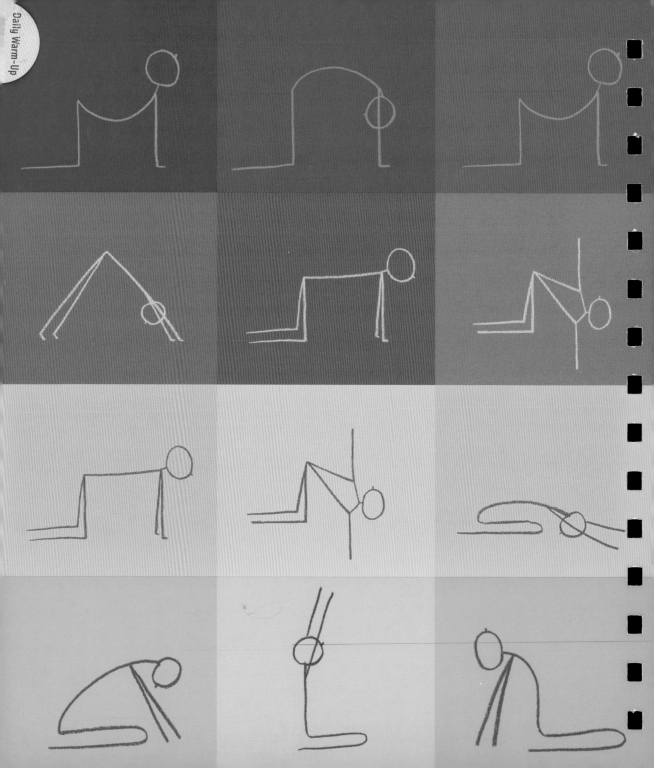

Daily Warm-Up

The daily warm-up is a short sequence of movements called a *vinyasa* or flow series. Each movement has a corresponding breath—inhale or exhale—that initiates the direction and energy of the movement. Because of the relationship between breath and movement, this flowing form creates heat, develops gracefulness and coordination, expands lung capacity, and cultivates mindfulness.

The inhalation relates to getting taller, extending out into space, filling up with air, and to *prana*, the life force. The exhalation is letting go, falling back into the center, softening, regenerating. We need both these directions to be complete. Try to make your inhalation and your exhalation equal in length as you begin to move through this *vinyasa* sequence. Notice when you are holding your breath. Don't worry about it, but simply breathe and keep going.

Since you will be doing this *vinyasa* every day, you will begin to get quite skillful at it. If you get bored with it, that's OK. Do it again and begin to pay more attention to what it feels like that day. You will find that although it's the same series of movements day in and day out, you are different every day. What you had for breakfast, what's going on at work, how well you slept, if your kids are sick—all these elements are part of your physical and mental experience.

Notice how your body is today—sluggish, strong, fluid? Notice how your mind is today—distracted, bored, upbeat? It's all fine. Do your practice no matter what. The practice of yoga is not about trying to be different from who you are, but rather understanding that we all have many aspects and that we are vast enough to contain numerous emotions and qualities. What does it feel like to be you right now?

The *vinyasa* form will also be incorporated into each day's special focus (for example, Wednesday, balancing poses), but first begin each practice with this warm-up. The sequence is designed to loosen up your entire spine, including your neck, which in turn will energize the entire body. It will also open your hip and shoulder joints, wrist and ankles, and elbows and knees and get you ready for the day's practice.

The daily warm-up sequence will take you approximately ninety seconds to do once. I recommend that you try to do it four times in a row. It is designed as a loop so that you can easily move back into the first asana (cow) from the last one (side bend to the right).

Daily Warm-Up

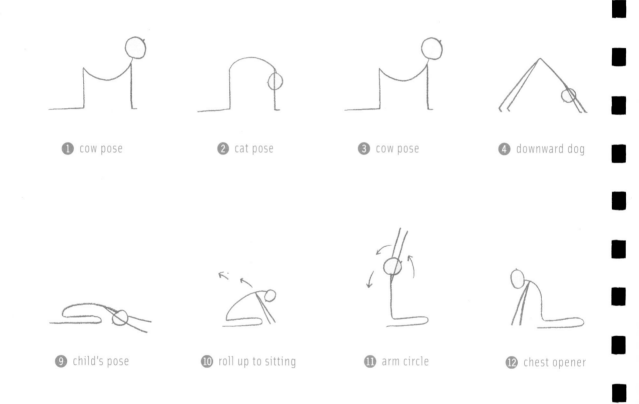

1. cow pose
2. cat pose
3. cow pose
4. downward dog

9. child's pose
10. roll up to sitting
11. arm circle
12. chest opener

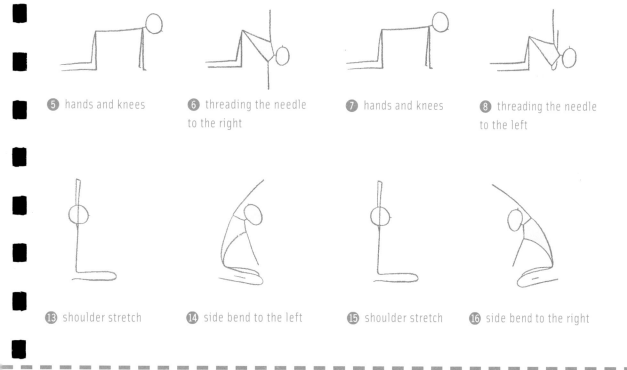

⑤ hands and knees

⑥ threading the needle to the right

⑦ hands and knees

⑧ threading the needle to the left

⑬ shoulder stretch

⑭ side bend to the left

⑮ shoulder stretch

⑯ side bend to the right

Do this sequence four times in a row. It is designed as a loop so that you can easily move back into the first asana (cow) from the last one (side bend to the right).

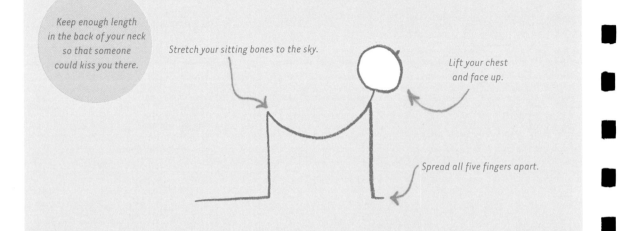

Keep enough length in the back of your neck so that someone could kiss you there.

Stretch your sitting bones to the sky.

Lift your chest and face up.

Spread all five fingers apart.

① cow pose

③ cow pose

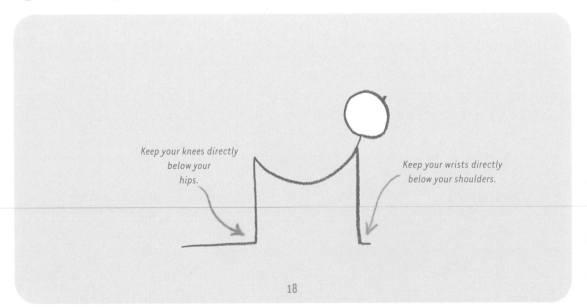

Keep your knees directly below your hips.

Keep your wrists directly below your shoulders.

18

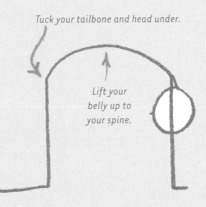

Tuck your tailbone and head under.

Lift your belly up to your spine.

2 cat pose

4 downward dog pose

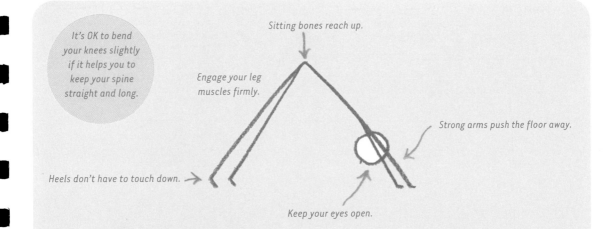

It's OK to bend your knees slightly if it helps you to keep your spine straight and long.

Sitting bones reach up.

Engage your leg muscles firmly.

Strong arms push the floor away.

Heels don't have to touch down. →

Keep your eyes open.

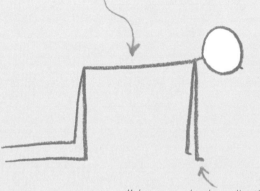

Find the length in your spine, from the tailbone to the crown of your head.

Make sure your hands are directly below your shoulders.

⑤ hands and knees

⑦ hands and knees

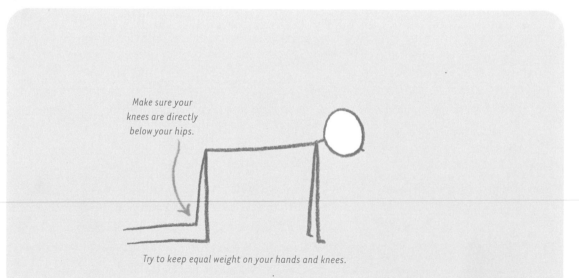

Make sure your knees are directly below your hips.

Try to keep equal weight on your hands and knees.

Spin your belly to the right and up.

Reach your right arm up and lengthen every single finger.

Make sure your hips don't move.
Twist at the waist, which will massage
and nourish your abdominal organs.

Extend your left shoulder and arm along the floor.

6 threading the needle to the right

8 threading the needle to the left

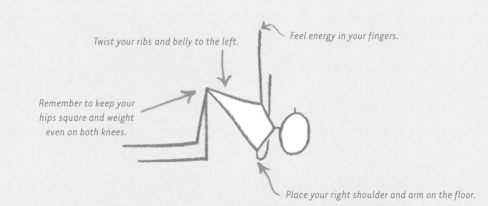

Twist your ribs and belly to the left.

Feel energy in your fingers.

Remember to keep your
hips square and weight
even on both knees.

Place your right shoulder and arm on the floor.

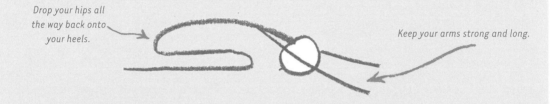

Feel your deep, full breath moving your back muscles.

Drop your hips all the way back onto your heels.

Keep your arms strong and long.

⑨ child's pose

⑪ arm circle

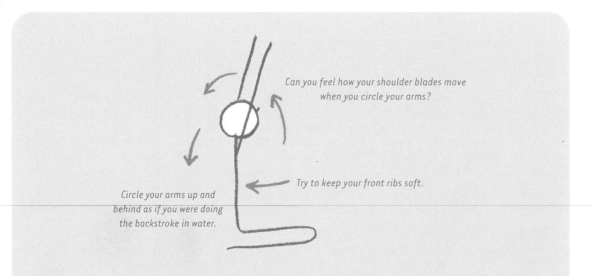

Can you feel how your shoulder blades move when you circle your arms?

Try to keep your front ribs soft.

Circle your arms up and behind as if you were doing the backstroke in water.

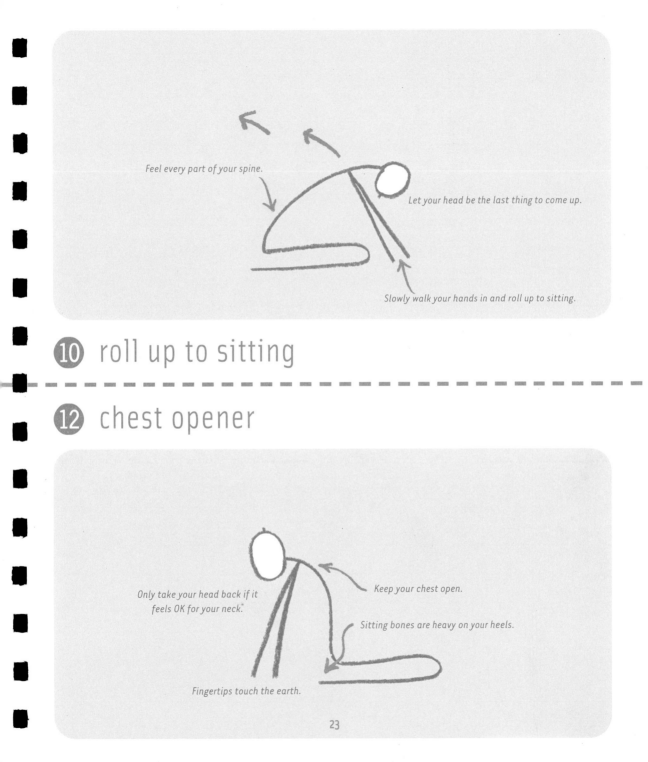

Feel every part of your spine.

Let your head be the last thing to come up.

Slowly walk your hands in and roll up to sitting.

⑩ roll up to sitting

⑫ chest opener

Only take your head back if it
feels OK for your neck.

Keep your chest open.

Sitting bones are heavy on your heels.

Fingertips touch the earth.

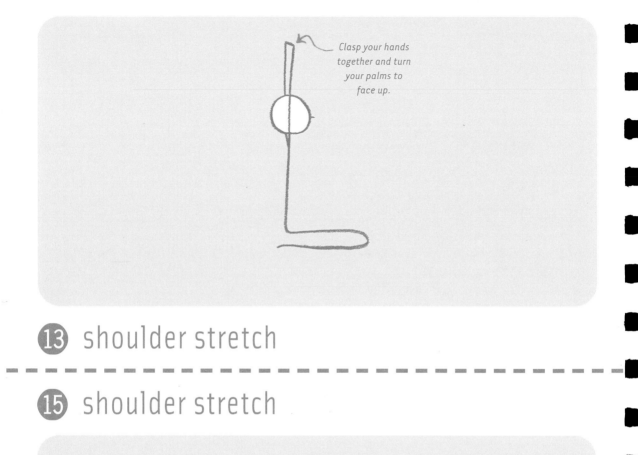

Clasp your hands together and turn your palms to face up.

⑬ shoulder stretch

---

⑮ shoulder stretch

Try to initiate the lift of the arms from the bottom of the ribs.

Open your right rib cage and feel it move with your breathing, like an accordion.

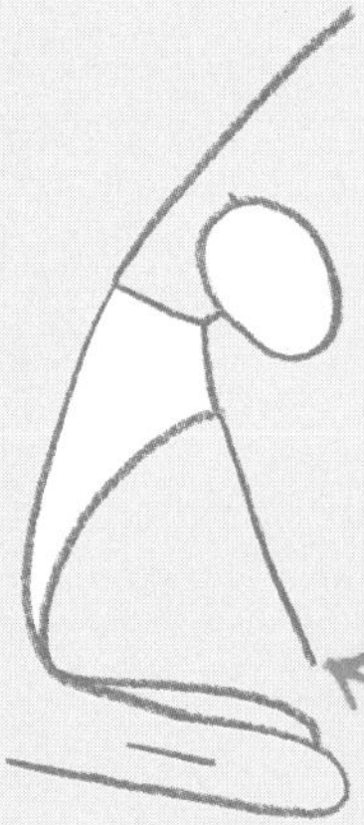

If sitting on your heels hurts your feet, put a blanket under you; if it hurts the back of your knees, put a blanket between your calves and thighs.

Left fingertips touch the floor.

⑭ side bend to the left

⑯ side bend to the right

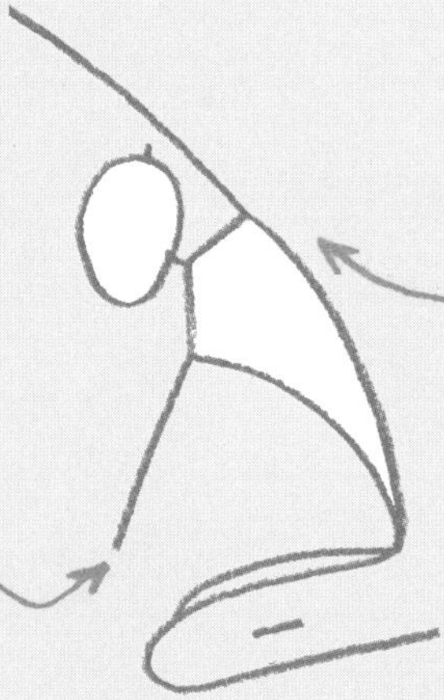

Really lengthen the whole left side of your body.

Place your right fingertips on the floor.

Daily Relaxation

At the end of every yoga class we rest by lying on our backs, with eyes closed. This is called corpse pose. In this pose we let go of all physical effort, including any special breathing techniques, and simply relax. You will notice that even though your body is still, your mind might be quite active. Don't try to push thoughts away. Without getting caught up in the contents of your mind, try simply to observe your thoughts coming into focus and fading away.

After five to ten minutes, begin to deepen your breathing again. Wiggle your toes and fingers. One at a time, bend your knees and place your feet on the floor. Roll onto your right side and rest there for a moment. Then, slowly, letting your head be the very last thing to come up, use your hands to walk your body back up to sitting. Place your cushion under your seat and stay there with your eyes closed for a few breaths.

Take a moment to see what it feels like to be you now. How is it different from the way you felt at the beginning of your session today? Chant Om three times.

You can also simply lay down flat on the ground and rest.

Cover up with a blanket if it's a chilly day.

Close your eyes.
An eye pillow can be nice.

Turn your palms up.

Feet should be about hip distance apart.

A pillow under your knees can feel good to your lower back.

corpse pose

side lying

After resting in corpse pose for five to ten minutes, roll onto your right side.

Rest here for a few moments. Use your hands to walk yourself back up to sitting. Gently curl up through your spine, with your head dangling. Let your head be the last thing to come up.

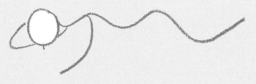

Dedicating Your Practice

After you chant Om three times at the end of your practice, take a few moments to absorb your experience. You may feel a sense of well-being, balance, spaciousness, even joy. These are the benefits of yoga, and they will begin to affect the "non-yoga" moments of your life as well.

You may notice these effects in small ways. Possibly you will not be so quick to get irritated by your kids. You may find that you are more patient with your coworkers or less judgmental of your spouse. These subtle but powerful changes will rub off on your friends and family so that their actions and attitudes may undergo a positive shift as well. In fact, our yoga practice of awakening will touch all our interactions, even those with strangers whom we normally don't even notice—the newspaper vendor, gas station attendant, dry cleaner—although we may see them daily.

Without even trying, our practice of balancing the body, resting the mind, and opening the heart will radiate out to the whole world. When we dedicate our practice we are consciously choosing to share these beneficial side effects of yoga with all the zillions of beings on the earth: those we love, those we don't love, those we feel neutral about, those we've never met, and of course, ourselves.

Here is a traditional Buddhist prayer that was taught to me by my teacher, Rimpoche Nawang Gehlek, which I say with my students at the end of every yoga class:

May all beings have happiness and the causes of happiness
May all beings be free from suffering and the causes of suffering
May all beings never be parted from freedom's true joy
May all beings dwell in equanimity free from attachment and aversion.

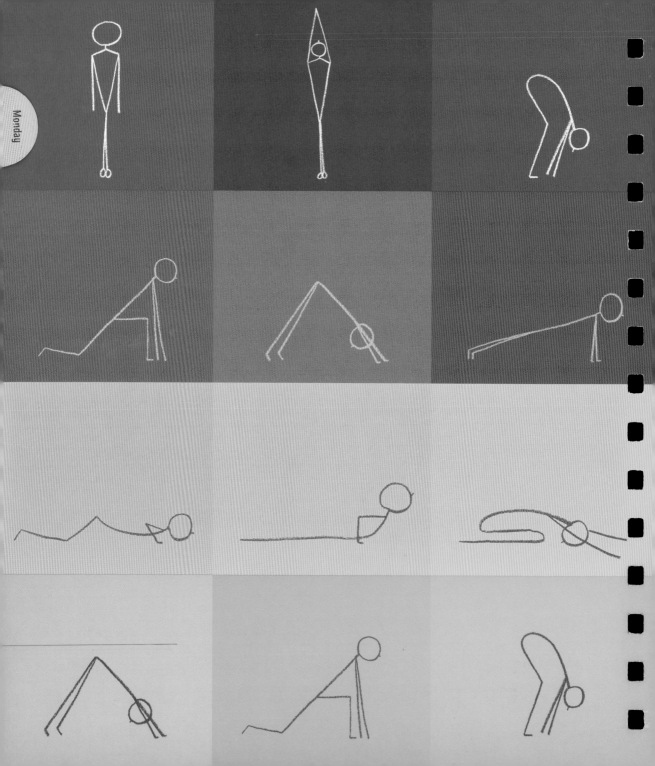

Monday

Monday

Saluting the sun is a traditional way for yogis to greet the day. Acknowledging the newness of each morning is a powerful reminder of the preciousness of our human lives and of our connection to nature.

The sun salute is a flowing sequence of alternating forward and backward bending movements that over time will generate physical stamina, strength, and mental focus.

I have noticed that my students have very high physical energy and strong motivation on Mondays. Our early-week pressures and eagerness can be harnessed and channeled through the robust physicality, steady breathing, and mindfulness of the sun salute series.

As you become more able to be precise in your movements and to breathe more smoothly, you will find that your mind becomes clear and spacious. Try to coordinate your arms and legs so that your entire body arrives in the pose at the same time.

It takes approximately forty-five seconds to do this *vinyasa*, but then you must do the sun salute sequence on the other side for a total of ninety seconds. I recommend that you repeat the sun salute on each side three times (right, left, right, left, right, left), which will take you about four and a half minutes.

Monday's Practice: Sun Salute

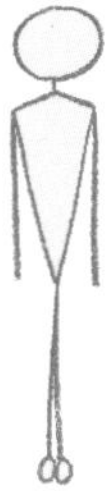

① mountain pose

② mountain pose arms up

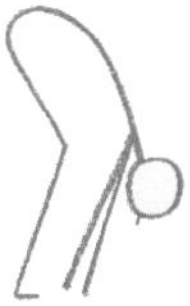

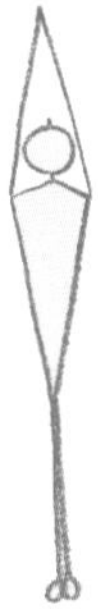

③ standing forward bend

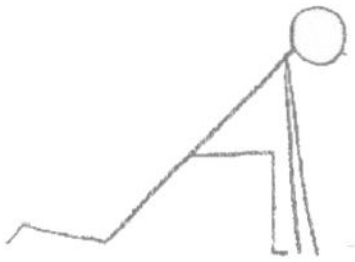

④ lunge, right leg back

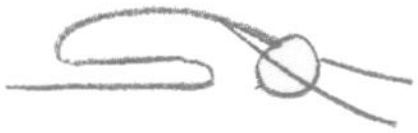

⑨ child's pose

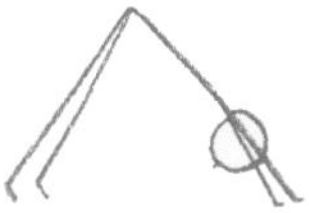

⑩ downward dog

⑪ lunge, right leg forward

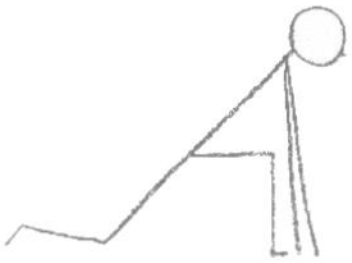

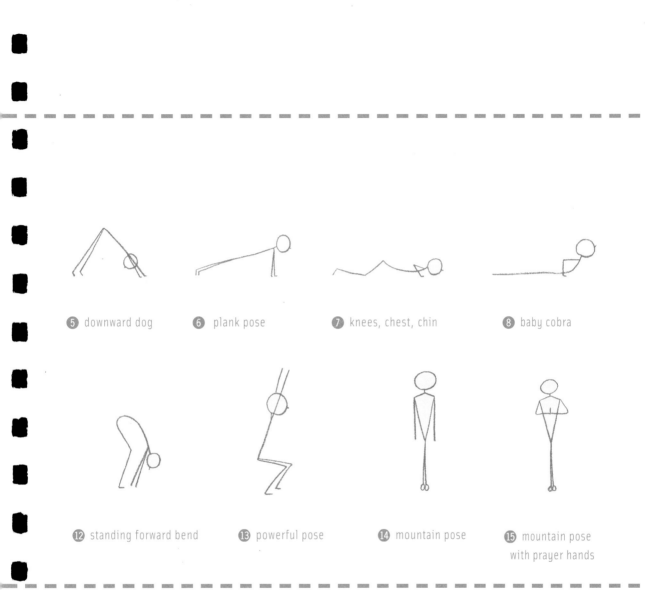

⑤ downward dog   ⑥ plank pose   ⑦ knees, chest, chin   ⑧ baby cobra

⑫ standing forward bend   ⑬ powerful pose   ⑭ mountain pose   ⑮ mountain pose with prayer hands

You must do this sequence two times, once beginning with the right leg and the second time with the left leg. I recommend that you repeat the sun salute on each side three times (right, left, right, left, right, left), which will take you about four and a half minutes.

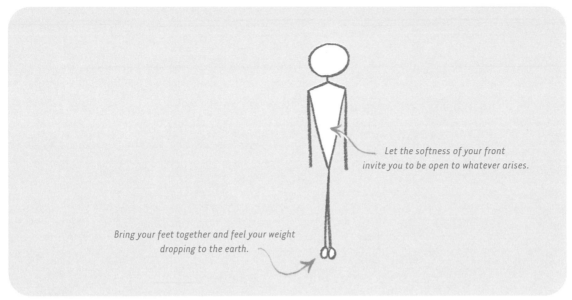

Let the softness of your front invite you to be open to whatever arises.

Bring your feet together and feel your weight dropping to the earth.

① mountain pose

③ standing forward bend

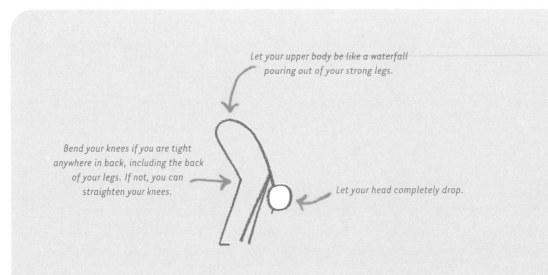

Let your upper body be like a waterfall pouring out of your strong legs.

Bend your knees if you are tight anywhere in back, including the back of your legs. If not, you can straighten your knees.

Let your head completely drop.

Press your palms together by
using your arm muscles.

Look up and see your palms meeting.

As you reach your arms up, reach your feet
down, so that your whole body lengthens
in two directions.

2 mountain pose arms up

4 lunge, right leg back

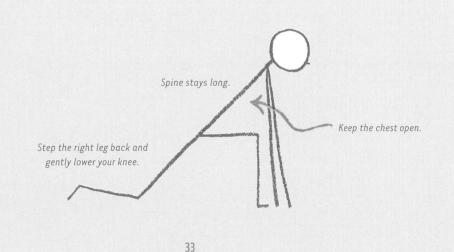

Spine stays long.

Keep the chest open.

Step the right leg back and
gently lower your knee.

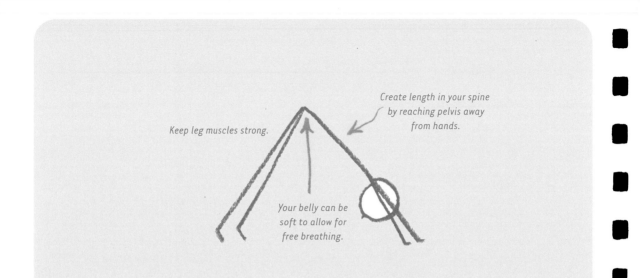

Create length in your spine by reaching pelvis away from hands.

Keep leg muscles strong.

Your belly can be soft to allow for free breathing.

⑤ downward dog

- -

⑦ knees, chest, chin

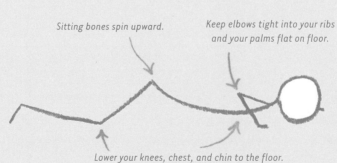

Sitting bones spin upward.

Keep elbows tight into your ribs and your palms flat on floor.

Lower your knees, chest, and chin to the floor.

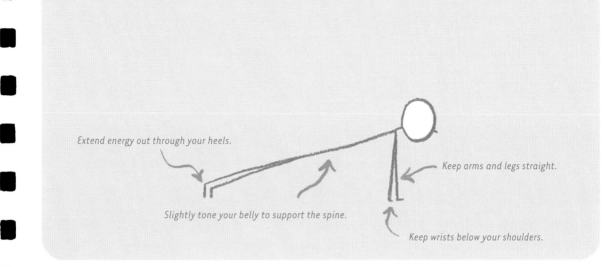

Extend energy out through your heels.

Keep arms and legs straight.

Slightly tone your belly to support the spine.

Keep wrists below your shoulders.

⑥ plank pose

⑧ baby cobra

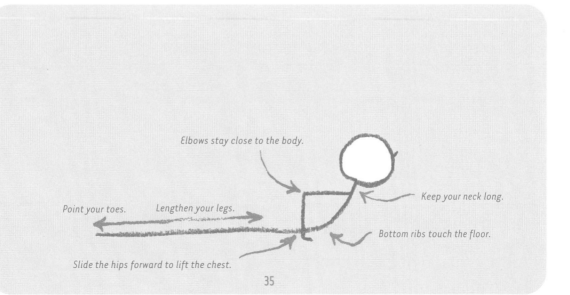

Elbows stay close to the body.

Keep your neck long.

Point your toes.   Lengthen your legs.

Bottom ribs touch the floor.

Slide the hips forward to lift the chest.

35

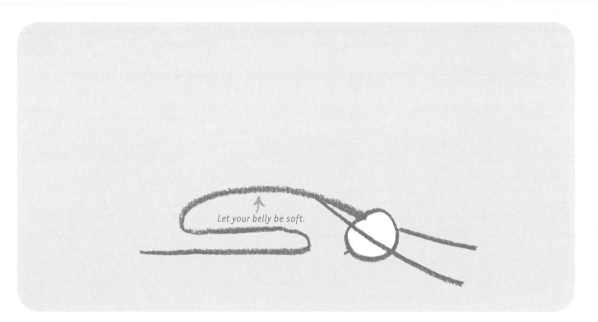

Let your belly be soft.

9 child's pose

11 lunge, right leg forward

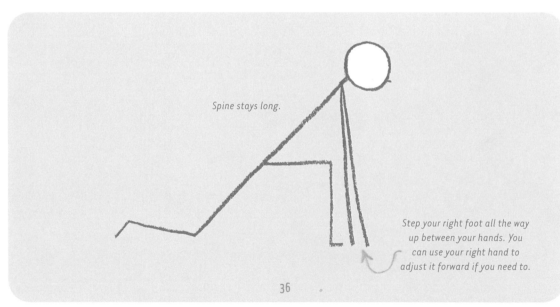

Spine stays long.

Step your right foot all the way up between your hands. You can use your right hand to adjust it forward if you need to.

Hold this downward facing dog for three to five breaths. A breath means one complete inhale and exhale.

Create length in your spine by reaching pelvis away from hands.

⑩ downward dog

----

⑫ standing forward bend

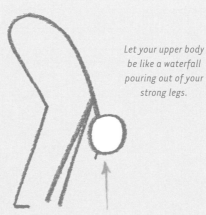

Let your upper body be like a waterfall pouring out of your strong legs.

Let your head completely drop.

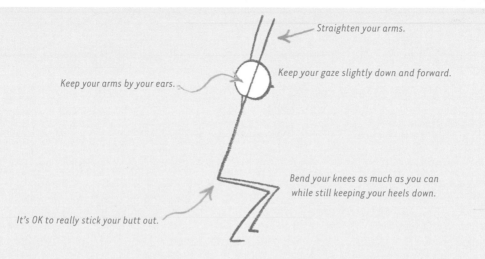

Straighten your arms.

Keep your gaze slightly down and forward.

Keep your arms by your ears.

Bend your knees as much as you can while still keeping your heels down.

It's OK to really stick your butt out.

13 powerful pose

14 mountain pose

Reach up to heaven with the crown of your head.

15 mountain pose with prayer hands

Let your tongue drop to the bottom of your mouth.

Close your eyes. Soften your face and throat.

Feel the movement of your heartbeat.

Feel the heat of your palms touching each other.

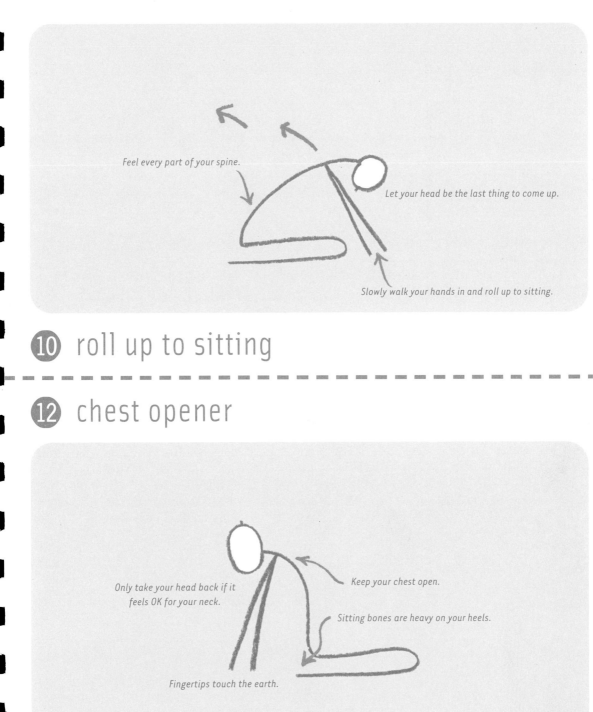

Feel every part of your spine.

Let your head be the last thing to come up.

Slowly walk your hands in and roll up to sitting.

⑩ roll up to sitting

⑫ chest opener

Only take your head back if it feels OK for your neck.

Keep your chest open.

Sitting bones are heavy on your heels.

Fingertips touch the earth.

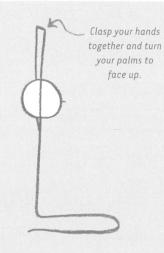

Clasp your hands together and turn your palms to face up.

⑬ shoulder stretch

---

⑮ shoulder stretch

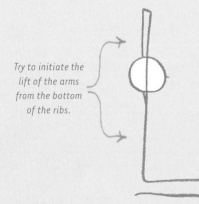

Try to initiate the lift of the arms from the bottom of the ribs.

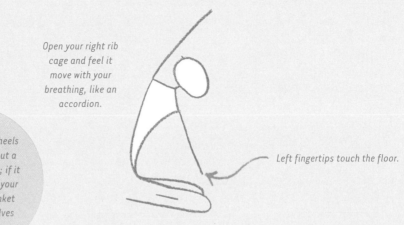

Open your right rib cage and feel it move with your breathing, like an accordion.

If sitting on your heels hurts your feet, put a blanket under you; if it hurts the back of your knees, put a blanket between your calves and thighs.

Left fingertips touch the floor.

⑭ side bend to the left

⑯ side bend to the right

Really lengthen the whole left side of your body.

Place your right fingertips on the floor.

Daily Relaxation

At the end of every yoga class we rest by lying on our backs, with eyes closed. This is called corpse pose. In this pose we let go of all physical effort, including any special breathing techniques, and simply relax. You will notice that even though your body is still, your mind might be quite active. Don't try to push thoughts away. Without getting caught up in the contents of your mind, try simply to observe your thoughts coming into focus and fading away.

After five to ten minutes, begin to deepen your breathing again. Wiggle your toes and fingers. One at a time, bend your knees and place your feet on the floor. Roll onto your right side and rest there for a moment. Then, slowly, letting your head be the very last thing to come up, use your hands to walk your body back up to sitting. Place your cushion under your seat and stay there with your eyes closed for a few breaths.

Take a moment to see what it feels like to be you now. How is it different from the way you felt at the beginning of your session today? Chant Om three times.

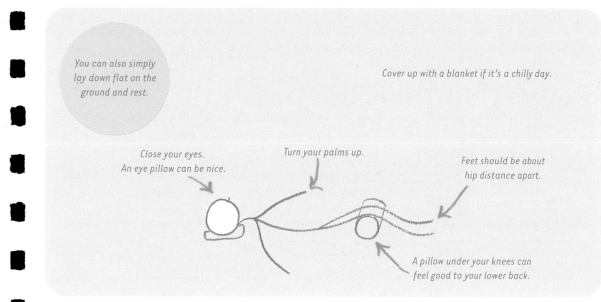

You can also simply lay down flat on the ground and rest.

Cover up with a blanket if it's a chilly day.

Close your eyes. An eye pillow can be nice.

Turn your palms up.

Feet should be about hip distance apart.

A pillow under your knees can feel good to your lower back.

corpse pose

side lying

After resting in corpse pose for five to ten minutes, roll onto your right side.

Rest here for a few moments. Use your hands to walk yourself back up to sitting. Gently curl up through your spine, with your head dangling. Let your head be the last thing to come up.

27

Dedicating Your Practice

After you chant Om three times at the end of your practice, take a few moments to absorb your experience. You may feel a sense of well-being, balance, spaciousness, even joy. These are the benefits of yoga, and they will begin to affect the "non-yoga" moments of your life as well.

You may notice these effects in small ways. Possibly you will not be so quick to get irritated by your kids. You may find that you are more patient with your coworkers or less judgmental of your spouse. These subtle but powerful changes will rub off on your friends and family so that their actions and attitudes may undergo a positive shift as well. In fact, our yoga practice of awakening will touch all our interactions, even those with strangers whom we normally don't even notice—the newspaper vendor, gas station attendant, dry cleaner—although we may see them daily.

Without even trying, our practice of balancing the body, resting the mind, and opening the heart will radiate out to the whole world. When we dedicate our practice we are consciously choosing to share these beneficial side effects of yoga with all the zillions of beings on the earth: those we love, those we don't love, those we feel neutral about, those we've never met, and of course, ourselves.

Here is a traditional Buddhist prayer that was taught to me by my teacher, Rimpoche Nawang Gehlek, which I say with my students at the end of every yoga class:

May all beings have happiness and the causes of happiness
May all beings be free from suffering and the causes of suffering
May all beings never be parted from freedom's true joy
May all beings dwell in equanimity free from attachment and aversion.

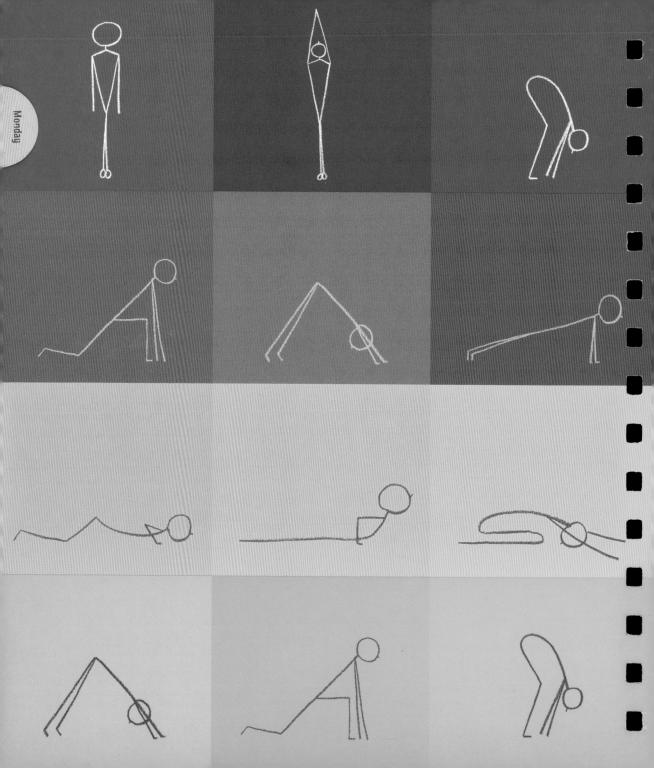

Monday

Saluting the sun is a traditional way for yogis to greet the day. Acknowledging the newness of each morning is a powerful reminder of the preciousness of our human lives and of our connection to nature.

The sun salute is a flowing sequence of alternating forward and backward bending movements that over time will generate physical stamina, strength, and mental focus.

I have noticed that my students have very high physical energy and strong motivation on Mondays. Our early-week pressures and eagerness can be harnessed and channeled through the robust physicality, steady breathing, and mindfulness of the sun salute series.

As you become more able to be precise in your movements and to breathe more smoothly, you will find that your mind becomes clear and spacious. Try to coordinate your arms and legs so that your entire body arrives in the pose at the same time.

It takes approximately forty-five seconds to do this *vinyasa*, but then you must do the sun salute sequence on the other side for a total of ninety seconds. I recommend that you repeat the sun salute on each side three times (right, left, right, left, right, left), which will take you about four and a half minutes.

Monday's Practice: Sun Salute

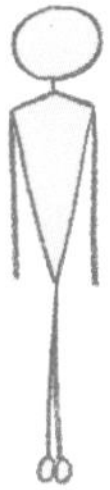

1 mountain pose

2 mountain pose arms up

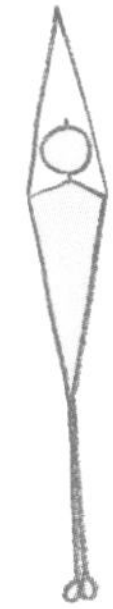

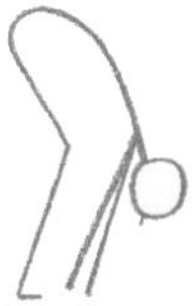

3 standing forward bend

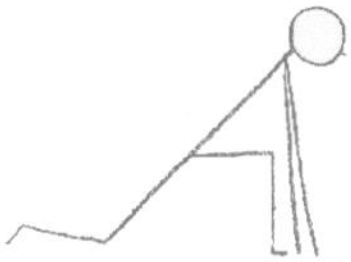

4 lunge, right leg back

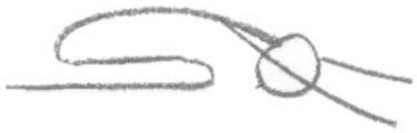

9 child's pose

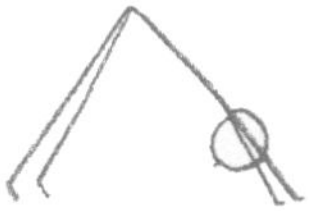

10 downward dog

11 lunge, right leg forward

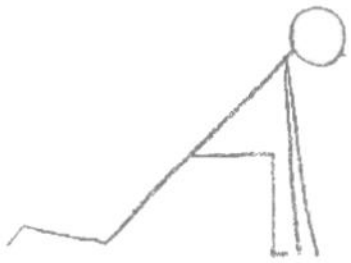

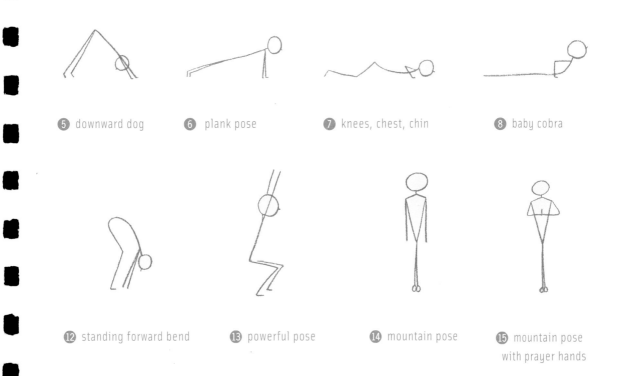

5 downward dog   6 plank pose   7 knees, chest, chin   8 baby cobra

12 standing forward bend   13 powerful pose   14 mountain pose   15 mountain pose with prayer hands

You must do this sequence two times, once beginning with the right leg and the second time with the left leg. I recommend that you repeat the sun salute on each side three times (right, left, right, left, right, left), which will take you about four and a half minutes.

Let the softness of your front
invite you to be open to whatever arises.

Bring your feet together and feel your weight
dropping to the earth.

1 mountain pose

3 standing forward bend

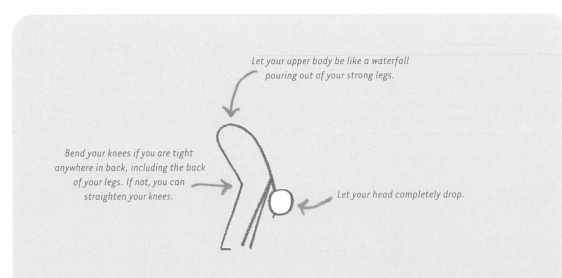

Let your upper body be like a waterfall
pouring out of your strong legs.

Bend your knees if you are tight
anywhere in back, including the back
of your legs. If not, you can
straighten your knees.

Let your head completely drop.

Press your palms together by
using your arm muscles.

Look up and see your palms meeting.

As you reach your arms up, reach your feet
down, so that your whole body lengthens
in two directions.

2 mountain pose arms up

4 lunge, right leg back

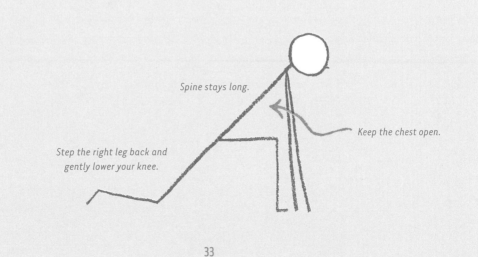

Spine stays long.

Keep the chest open.

Step the right leg back and
gently lower your knee.

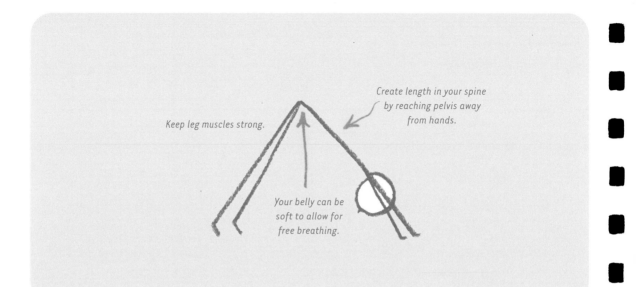

Create length in your spine by reaching pelvis away from hands.

Keep leg muscles strong.

Your belly can be soft to allow for free breathing.

⑤ downward dog

⑦ knees, chest, chin

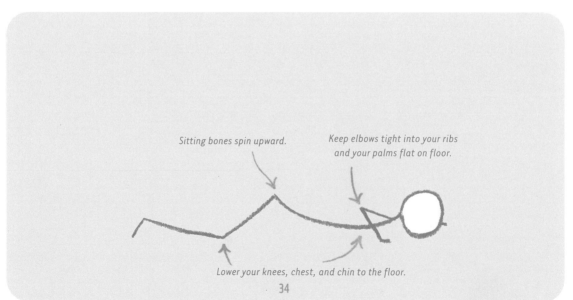

Sitting bones spin upward.

Keep elbows tight into your ribs and your palms flat on floor.

Lower your knees, chest, and chin to the floor.

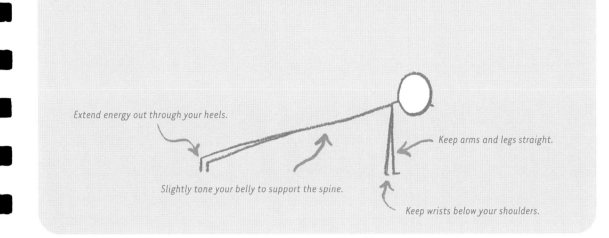

Extend energy out through your heels.

Keep arms and legs straight.

Slightly tone your belly to support the spine.

Keep wrists below your shoulders.

6 plank pose

8 baby cobra

Elbows stay close to the body.

Keep your neck long.

Point your toes.   Lengthen your legs.

Bottom ribs touch the floor.

Slide the hips forward to lift the chest.

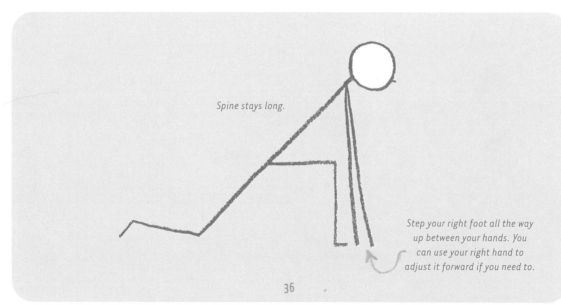

Let your belly be soft.

⑨ child's pose

---

⑪ lunge, right leg forward

Spine stays long.

Step your right foot all the way up between your hands. You can use your right hand to adjust it forward if you need to.

Hold this downward facing dog for three to five breaths. A breath means one complete inhale and exhale.

Create length in your spine by reaching pelvis away from hands.

⑩ downward dog

⑫ standing forward bend

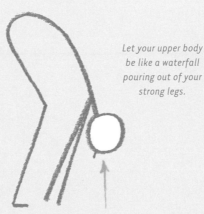

Let your upper body be like a waterfall pouring out of your strong legs.

Let your head completely drop.

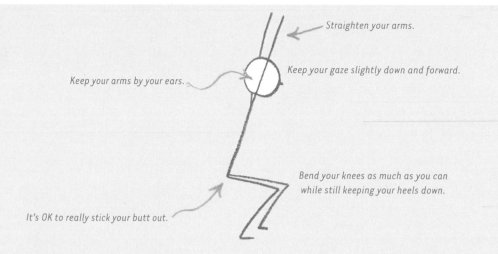

Straighten your arms.

Keep your gaze slightly down and forward.

Keep your arms by your ears.

Bend your knees as much as you can while still keeping your heels down.

It's OK to really stick your butt out.

13 powerful pose

14 mountain pose

Reach up to heaven with the crown of your head.

15 mountain pose with prayer hands

Let your tongue drop to the bottom of your mouth.

Close your eyes. Soften your face and throat.

Feel the movement of your heartbeat.

Feel the heat of your palms touching each other.

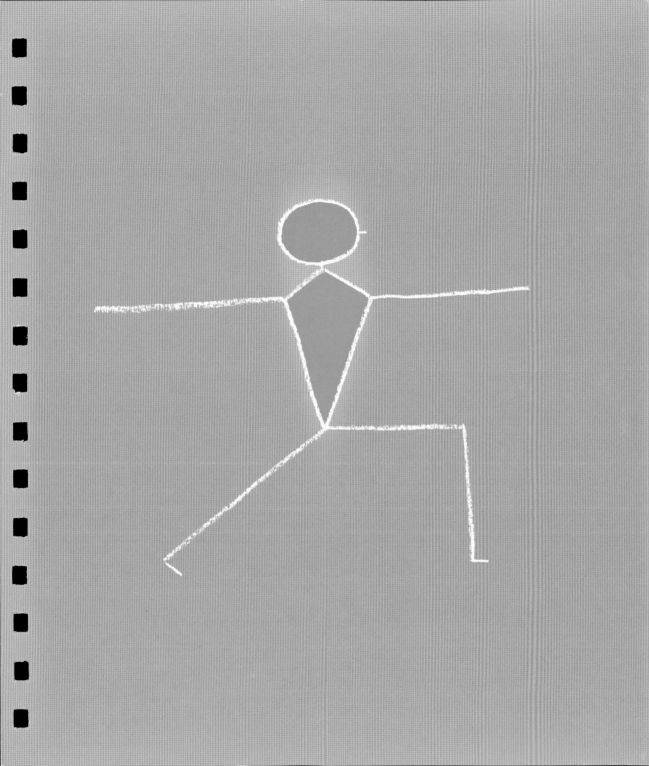

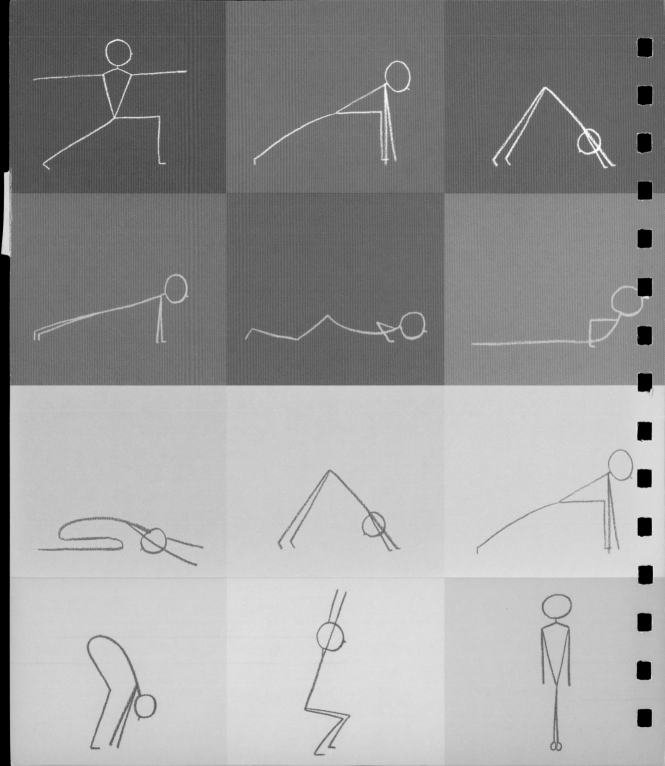

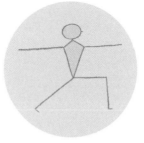

Tuesday

Standing poses are the best way to develop strength for everyday living—sitting, standing, walking, and laying down. The standing poses strengthen the arms and legs, considered the organs of action in yoga, and create proper alignment through the entire body. Once you begin to experience confidence in rooting your legs, you may begin to notice a corresponding uplift in your spine and heart. This feeling of connection—down to the earth and upward to heaven—helps us to feel more comfortable in our own bodies as we move through the world.

On Tuesdays my students usually still feel strong and motivated but somewhat more grounded, and that is an essential element in standing poses.

This standing pose sequence will take four minutes to complete both sides.

Tuesday's Practice: Standing Poses

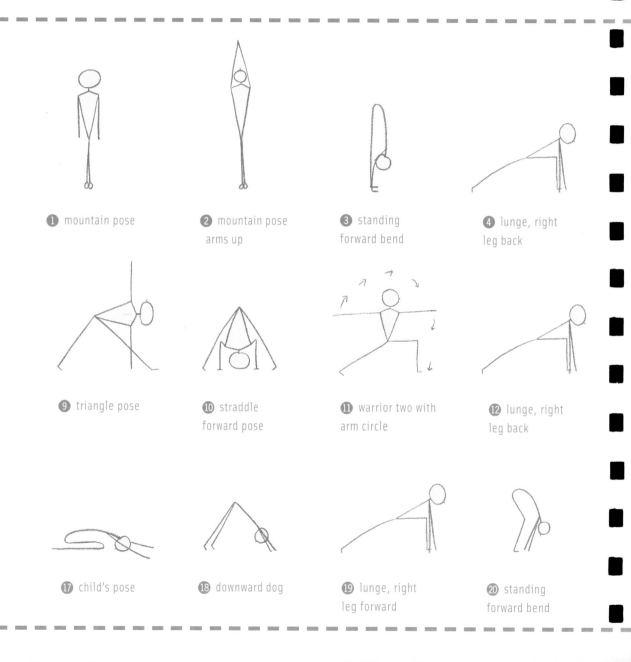

1 mountain pose

2 mountain pose arms up

3 standing forward bend

4 lunge, right leg back

9 triangle pose

10 straddle forward pose

11 warrior two with arm circle

12 lunge, right leg back

17 child's pose

18 downward dog

19 lunge, right leg forward

20 standing forward bend

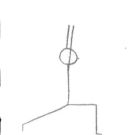
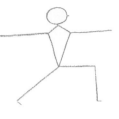
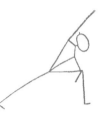
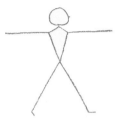

5 warrior one   **6** warrior two   **7** side-extended angle   **8** warrior two, straight legs

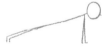
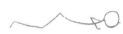

13 downward dog   **14** plank pose   **15** knees, chest, chin   **16** baby cobra

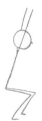
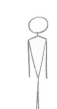

21 powerful pose   **22** mountain pose

This standing pose sequence must be done twice, once leading with the right leg, once leading with the left leg.

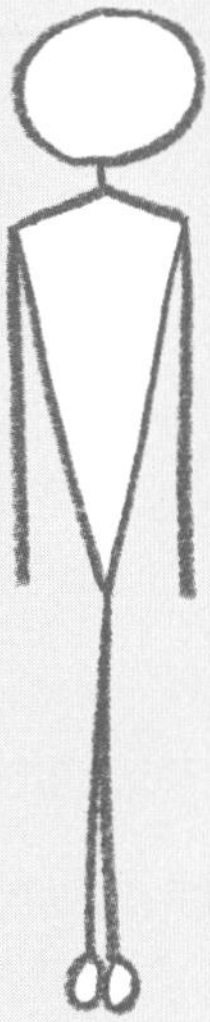

Let the strength of your back give you confidence.

1 mountain pose

- -

3 standing forward bend

Do not bounce or try to stretch your legs more. Instead, engage the leg muscles actively, breathe deeply, and cultivate patience.

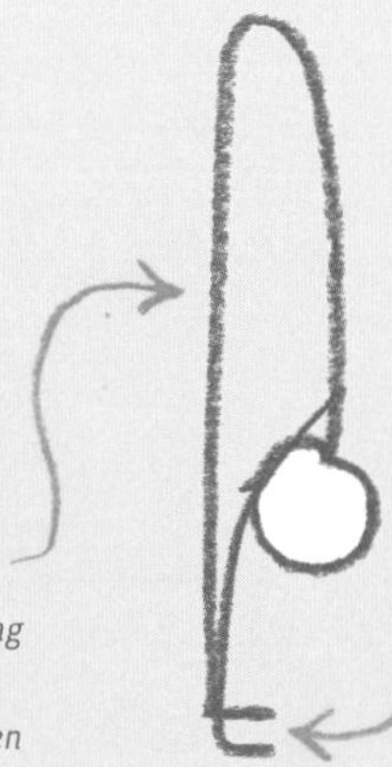

Extend your spine in two directions. Go for length rather than trying to touch your nose to your legs.

Bend your knees if you are tight anywhere on your back body, including the back of your legs. If not, you can straighten your knees.

Keep fingertips in line with toe tips.

42

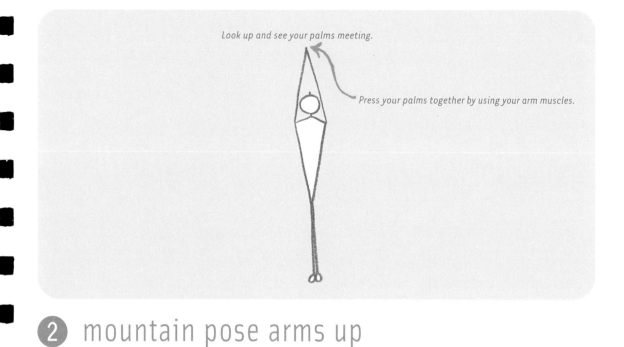

Look up and see your palms meeting.

Press your palms together by using your arm muscles.

② mountain pose arms up

④ lunge, right leg back

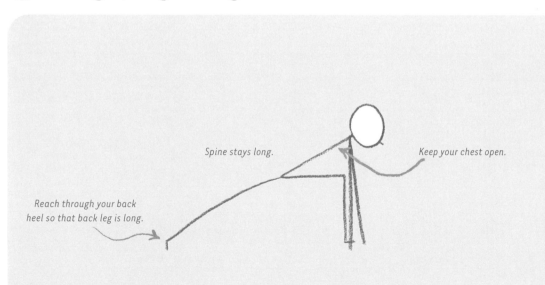

Spine stays long.

Keep your chest open.

Reach through your back heel so that back leg is long.

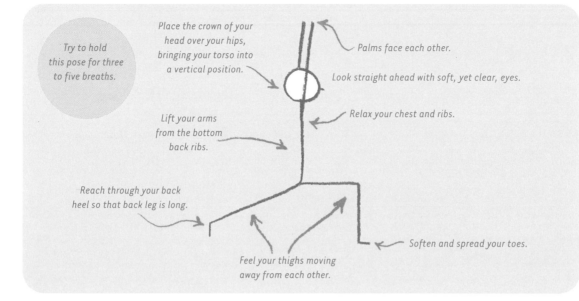

Try to hold this pose for three to five breaths.

Place the crown of your head over your hips, bringing your torso into a vertical position.

Palms face each other.

Look straight ahead with soft, yet clear, eyes.

Relax your chest and ribs.

Lift your arms from the bottom back ribs.

Reach through your back heel so that back leg is long.

Soften and spread your toes.

Feel your thighs moving away from each other.

⑤ warrior one

- -

⑦ side-extended angle

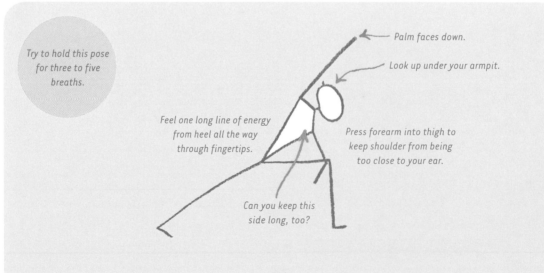

Try to hold this pose for three to five breaths.

Palm faces down.

Look up under your armpit.

Feel one long line of energy from heel all the way through fingertips.

Press forearm into thigh to keep shoulder from being too close to your ear.

Can you keep this side long, too?

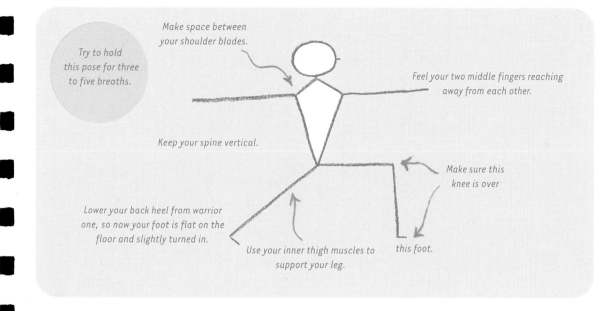

Make space between your shoulder blades.

Try to hold this pose for three to five breaths.

Feel your two middle fingers reaching away from each other.

Keep your spine vertical.

Make sure this knee is over

Lower your back heel from warrior one, so now your foot is flat on the floor and slightly turned in.

Use your inner thigh muscles to support your leg.

this foot.

6 warrior two

8 warrior two, straight legs

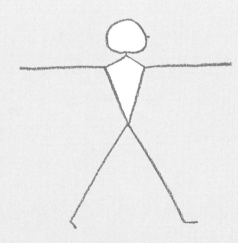

Stay in warrior two, only now keep both legs straight.

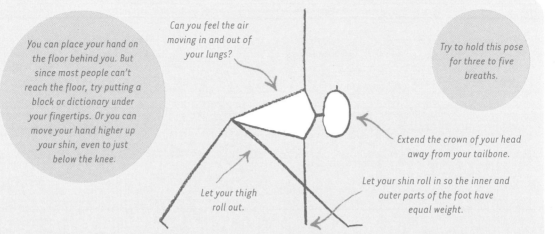

You can place your hand on the floor behind you. But since most people can't reach the floor, try putting a block or dictionary under your fingertips. Or you can move your hand higher up your shin, even to just below the knee.

Can you feel the air moving in and out of your lungs?

Try to hold this pose for three to five breaths.

Extend the crown of your head away from your tailbone.

Let your shin roll in so the inner and outer parts of the foot have equal weight.

Let your thigh roll out.

Reach down into the earth with this leg.

⑨ triangle pose

⑪ warrior two with arm circle

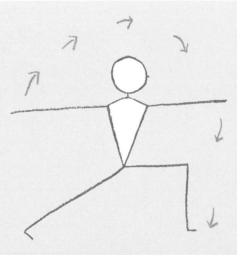

From straddle forward pose, place your hands on your waist and come up to standing on straight legs. Turn one leg out, coming back into warrior two.

•NOW•
Circle your back arm up and over, then place both arms on the floor on either side of your front foot.

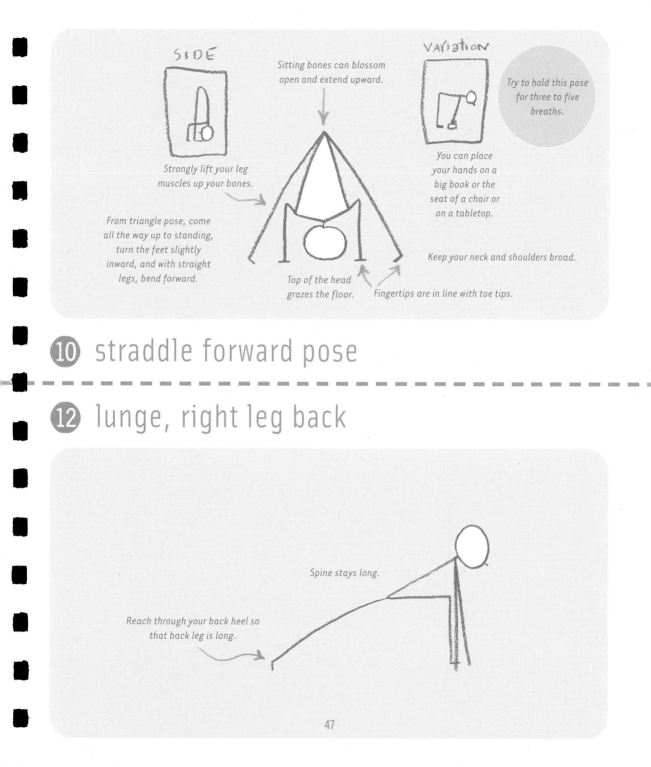

SIDE

Sitting bones can blossom
open and extend upward.

VARIATION

Try to hold this pose
for three to five
breaths.

Strongly lift your leg
muscles up your bones.

You can place
your hands on a
big book or the
seat of a chair or
on a tabletop.

From triangle pose, come
all the way up to standing,
turn the feet slightly
inward, and with straight
legs, bend forward.

Top of the head
grazes the floor.

Fingertips are in line with toe tips.

Keep your neck and shoulders broad.

⑩ straddle forward pose

⑫ lunge, right leg back

Spine stays long.

Reach through your back heel so
that back leg is long.

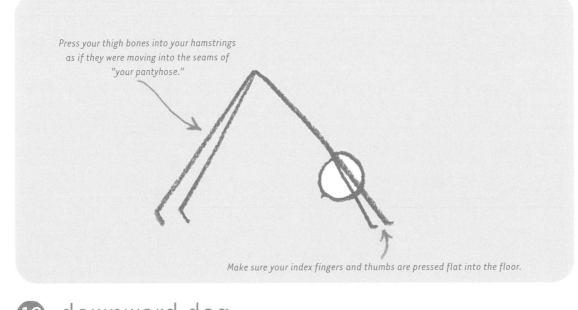

Press your thigh bones into your hamstrings as if they were moving into the seams of "your pantyhose."

Make sure your index fingers and thumbs are pressed flat into the floor.

⑬ downward dog

- -

⑮ knees chest chin

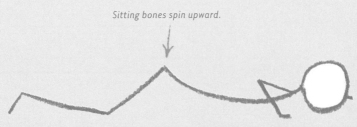

Keep your elbows tight against the ribs, and palms flat on the floor.

Sitting bones spin upward.

Lower your knees, chest, and chin to the floor.

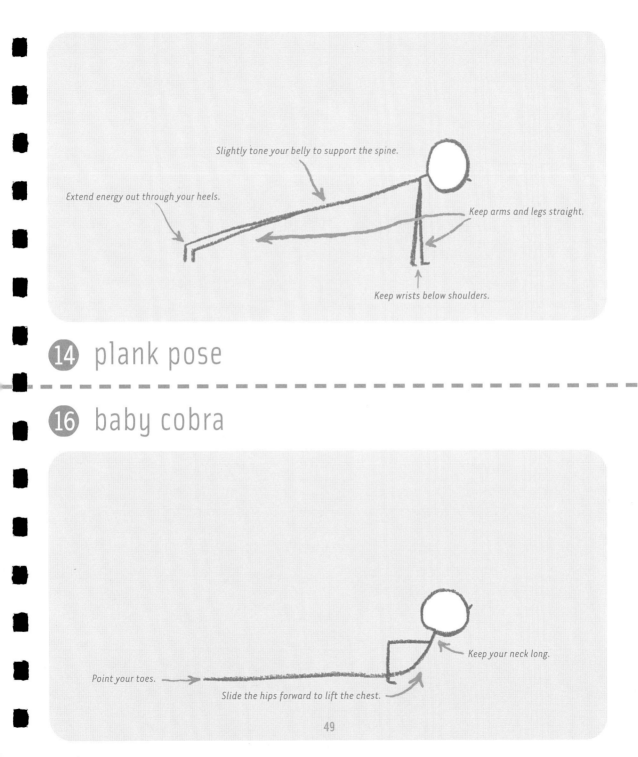

Slightly tone your belly to support the spine.

Extend energy out through your heels.

Keep arms and legs straight.

Keep wrists below shoulders.

14 plank pose

16 baby cobra

Point your toes.

Slide the hips forward to lift the chest.

Keep your neck long.

49

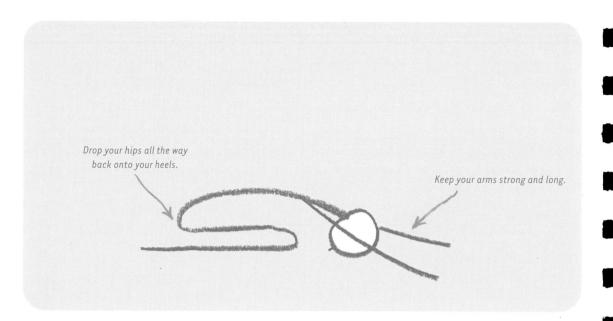

Drop your hips all the way
back onto your heels.

Keep your arms strong and long.

⑰ child's pose

⑲ lunge, right leg forward

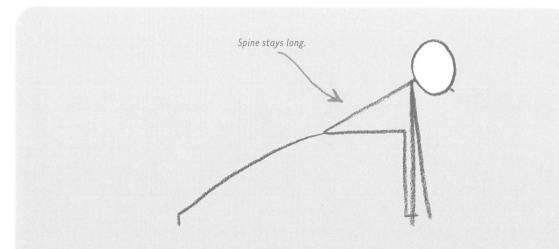

Spine stays long.

Step your right foot all the way up between your hands. You can use your right hand to adjust it forward if you need to.

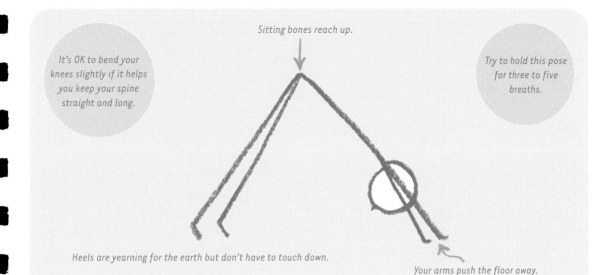

Sitting bones reach up.

It's OK to bend your knees slightly if it helps you keep your spine straight and long.

Try to hold this pose for three to five breaths.

Heels are yearning for the earth but don't have to touch down.

Your arms push the floor away.

18 downward dog

20 standing forward bend

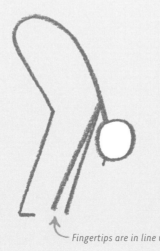

Do not bounce or try to stretch your legs more. Instead, engage the leg muscles actively, breathe deeply, and cultivate patience.

Fingertips are in line with toe tips.

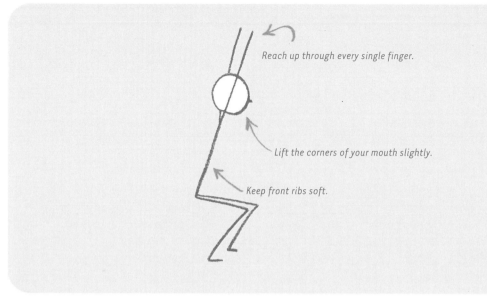

Reach up through every single finger.

Lift the corners of your mouth slightly.

Keep front ribs soft.

 powerful pose

 mountain pose

Let the softness of your front invite you to be open to whatever arises.

Bring your feet together and feel your weight dropping to the earth.

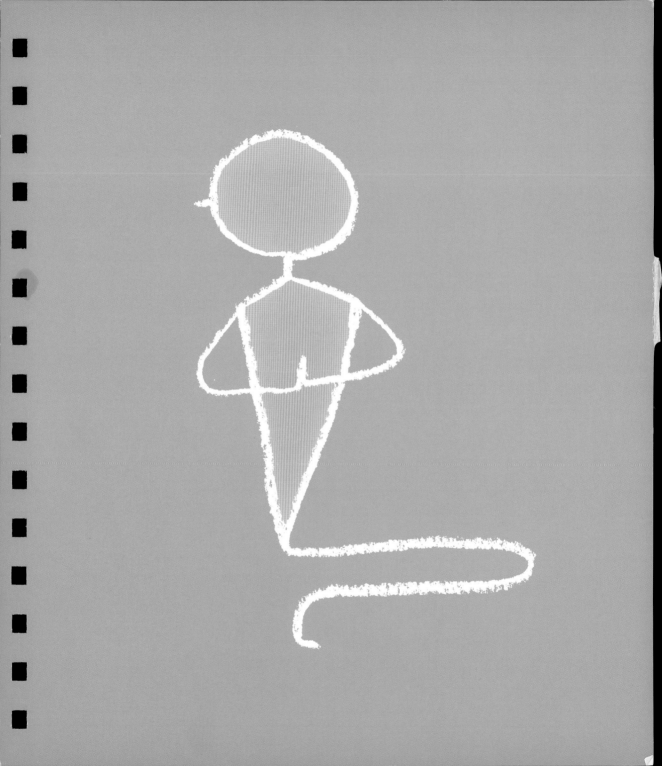

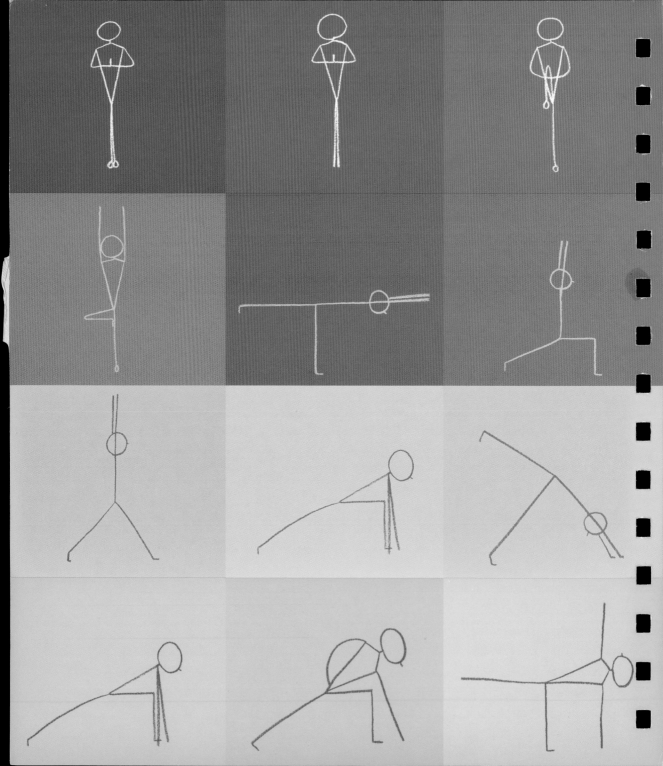

Wednesday

Wednesday is the perfect day to work on balancing, since it is halfway between the high energy of the beginning of the week and the relaxation and fun that await us on the weekend.

In this sequence of balancing poses, you will balance on two legs, on one leg, on two legs and one arm, and on one arm and one leg. You will work on balancing the front and back of your body, and your right and left sides, and on extending down through your legs and up through the crown of your head.

But balancing practice also involves balancing effort and release, stabilizing your mind, and finding equanimity with your breathing. Some of these poses are quite challenging, and at some point you will certainly fall over. Notice what comes up in your mind when that happens, and apply the meditation technique of labeling it "thinking" and letting it go.

See if you can discover any relationship among the activities of your mind, the movement of your breathing, and your ability to find physical balance. The challenges of these poses are nothing compared to your regular life, so consider this a practice session for staying centered when your life spins out of control or throws you for a loop.

The total time for this series is seven minutes.

Wednesday's Practice: Balancing Poses

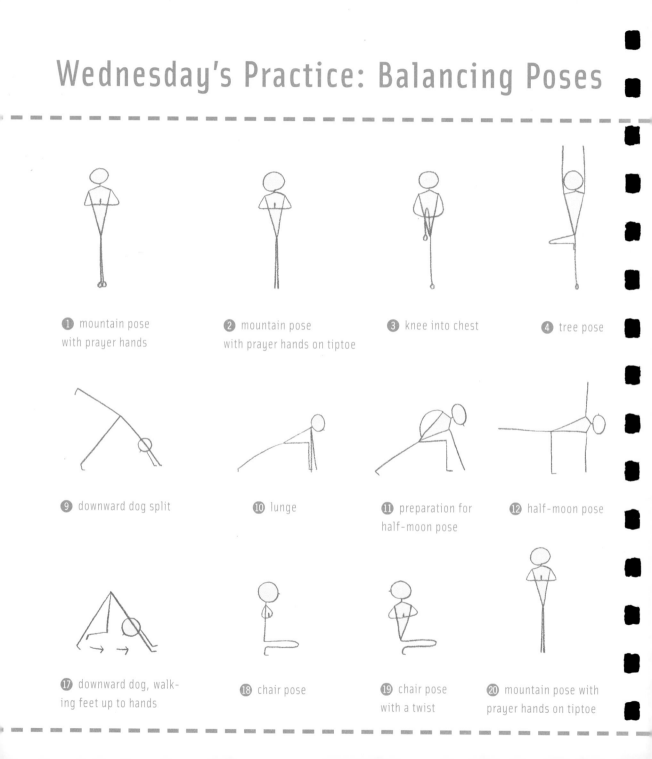

1 mountain pose with prayer hands

2 mountain pose with prayer hands on tiptoe

3 knee into chest

4 tree pose

9 downward dog split

10 lunge

11 preparation for half-moon pose

12 half-moon pose

17 downward dog, walking feet up to hands

18 chair pose

19 chair pose with a twist

20 mountain pose with prayer hands on tiptoe

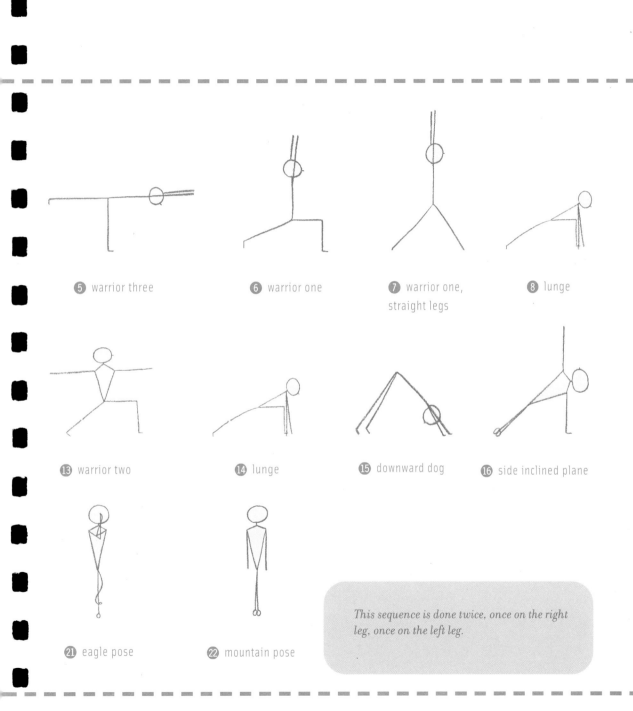

⑤ warrior three

⑥ warrior one

⑦ warrior one, straight legs

⑧ lunge

⑬ warrior two

⑭ lunge

⑮ downward dog

⑯ side inclined plane

㉑ eagle pose

㉒ mountain pose

This sequence is done twice, once on the right leg, once on the left leg.

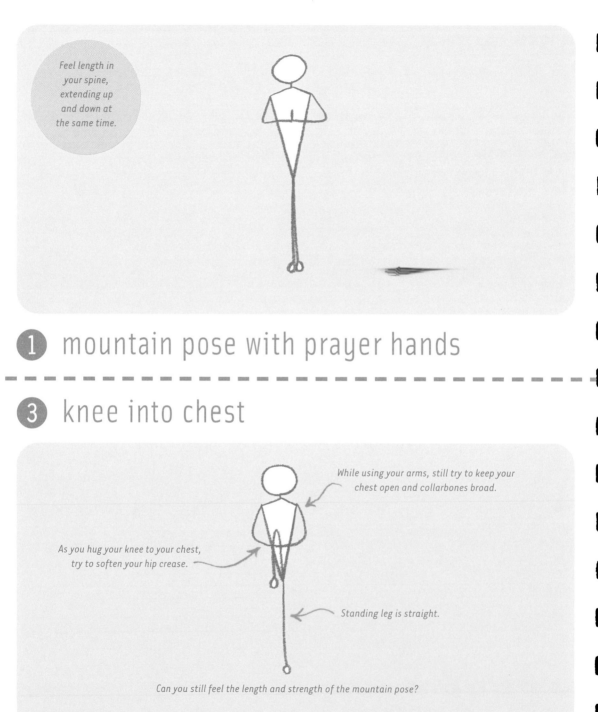

Feel length in your spine, extending up and down at the same time.

1 mountain pose with prayer hands

3 knee into chest

While using your arms, still try to keep your chest open and collarbones broad.

As you hug your knee to your chest, try to soften your hip crease.

Standing leg is straight.

Can you still feel the length and strength of the mountain pose?

Pick something at eye level and rest your gaze there. This will help you stay steady and balanced.

Feel length in your spine, extending up and down at the same time.

Repeat for three breaths in and out, rising up and down on the toes, three times.

Inhale and rise up on your toes. Exhale to lower down.

Squeeze your inner thighs together.

Bring your feet all the way together and press down with the balls of your toes as you lift your heels off the floor.

2 mountain pose with prayer hands on tiptoe

4 tree pose

Imagine that you are a tree and that the dirt is at your waist. Your legs are the roots, your spine is the trunk, and your arms are the branches.

Try to hold this pose for three to five breaths.

Keep both hip points facing forward like headlights.

Can you feel yourself rooting and rising at the same time?

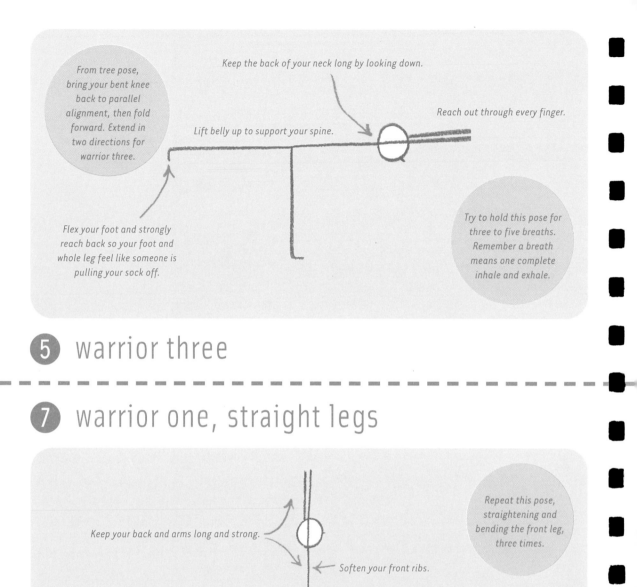

From tree pose, bring your bent knee back to parallel alignment, then fold forward. Extend in two directions for warrior three.

Keep the back of your neck long by looking down.

Reach out through every finger.

Lift belly up to support your spine.

Flex your foot and strongly reach back so your foot and whole leg feel like someone is pulling your sock off.

Try to hold this pose for three to five breaths. Remember a breath means one complete inhale and exhale.

5 warrior three

7 warrior one, straight legs

Keep your back and arms long and strong.

Repeat this pose, straightening and bending the front leg, three times.

Soften your front ribs.

Lift your knees and thigh muscles.

Press down into the floor to straighten your legs.

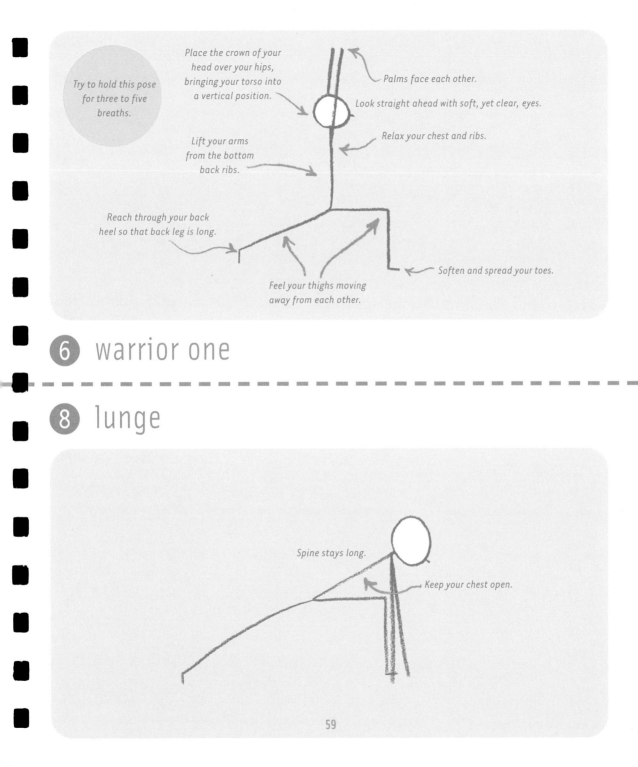

Try to hold this pose for three to five breaths.

Place the crown of your head over your hips, bringing your torso into a vertical position.

Palms face each other.

Look straight ahead with soft, yet clear, eyes.

Relax your chest and ribs.

Lift your arms from the bottom back ribs.

Reach through your back heel so that back leg is long.

Soften and spread your toes.

Feel your thighs moving away from each other.

⑥ warrior one

⑧ lunge

Spine stays long.

Keep your chest open.

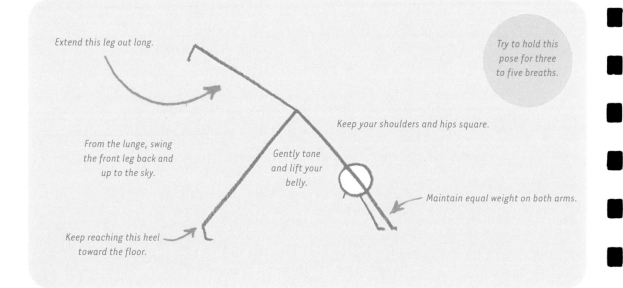

Extend this leg out long.

Try to hold this pose for three to five breaths.

Keep your shoulders and hips square.

From the lunge, swing the front leg back and up to the sky.

Gently tone and lift your belly.

Maintain equal weight on both arms.

Keep reaching this heel toward the floor.

⑨ downward dog split

- -

⑪ preparation for half-moon pose

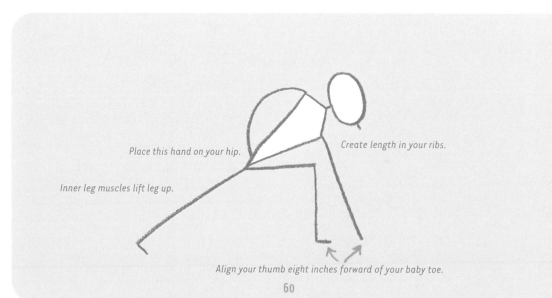

Place this hand on your hip.

Create length in your ribs.

Inner leg muscles lift leg up.

Align your thumb eight inches forward of your baby toe.

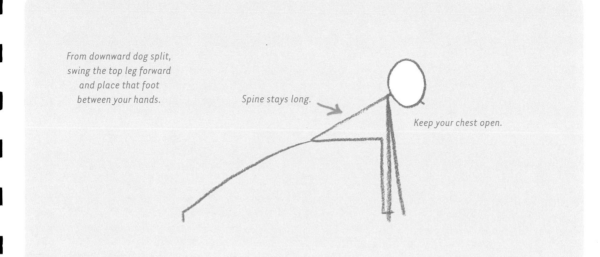

From downward dog split, swing the top leg forward and place that foot between your hands.

Spine stays long.

Keep your chest open.

10 lunge

12 half-moon pose

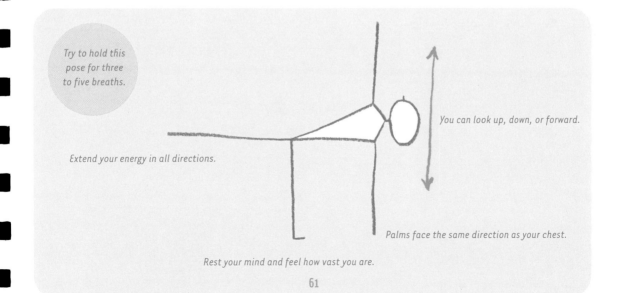

Try to hold this pose for three to five breaths.

You can look up, down, or forward.

Extend your energy in all directions.

Palms face the same direction as your chest.

Rest your mind and feel how vast you are.

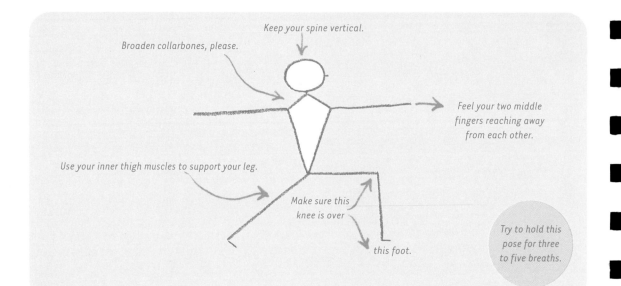

Keep your spine vertical.

Broaden collarbones, please.

Feel your two middle
fingers reaching away
from each other.

Use your inner thigh muscles to support your leg.

Make sure this
knee is over

this foot.

Try to hold this
pose for three
to five breaths.

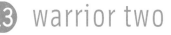

⑬ warrior two

⑮ downward dog

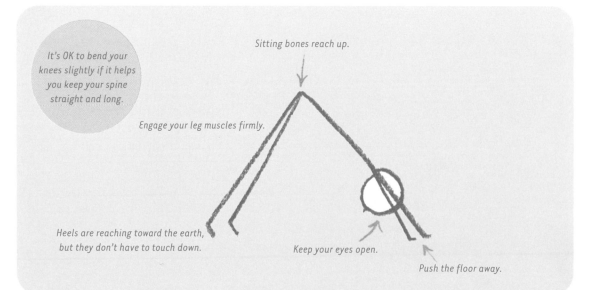

It's OK to bend your
knees slightly if it helps
you keep your spine
straight and long.

Sitting bones reach up.

Engage your leg muscles firmly.

Heels are reaching toward the earth,
but they don't have to touch down.

Keep your eyes open.

Push the floor away.

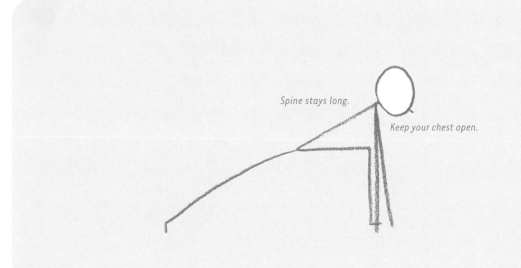

Spine stays long.

Keep your chest open.

⑭ lunge

⑯ side inclined plane

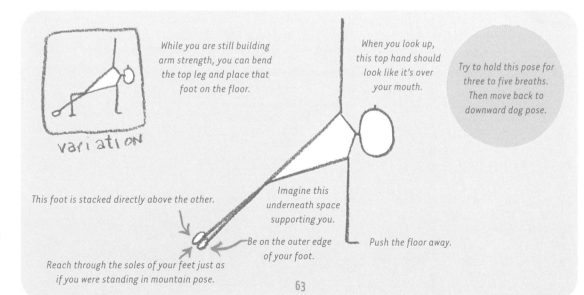

variation

While you are still building arm strength, you can bend the top leg and place that foot on the floor.

When you look up, this top hand should look like it's over your mouth.

Try to hold this pose for three to five breaths. Then move back to downward dog pose.

This foot is stacked directly above the other.

Imagine this underneath space supporting you.

Be on the outer edge of your foot.

Push the floor away.

Reach through the soles of your feet just as if you were standing in mountain pose.

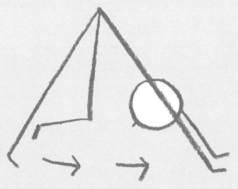

Slowly walk your feet to your hands as if you were doing a walking meditation. Feel the texture of the floor as you move toe, ball, heel.

Bend your knees however you need to.

⑰ downward dog, walking feet up to hands

⑲ chair pose with a twist

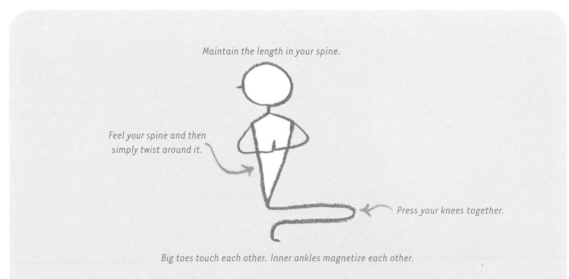

Maintain the length in your spine.

Feel your spine and then simply twist around it.

Press your knees together.

Big toes touch each other. Inner ankles magnetize each other.

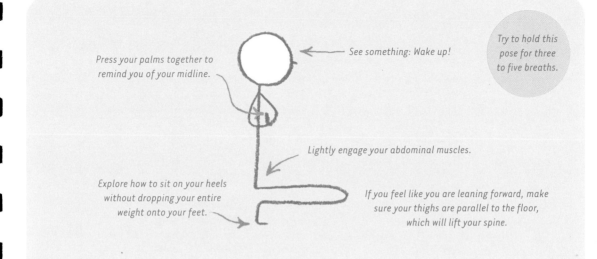

Press your palms together to remind you of your midline.

See something: Wake up!

Try to hold this pose for three to five breaths.

Lightly engage your abdominal muscles.

Explore how to sit on your heels without dropping your entire weight onto your feet.

If you feel like you are leaning forward, make sure your thighs are parallel to the floor, which will lift your spine.

18 chair pose

20 mountain pose with prayer hands on tiptoe

Pick something at eye level and rest your gaze there to stay steady and balanced.

Squeeze your inner thighs together.

Bring your feet all the way together and press down with the balls of your toes as you lift your heels off the floor.

Place one upper arm over the other, then cross your wrists and press your palms together. If you can't reach your palms together, don't cross your wrists, but simply touch the backs of your hands together.

Let your gaze be panoramic. Even see out the back of your head.

The arm that wraps on top should be the opposite of the leg that is on top.

This is always a wibbly-wobbly balance. Just try to stay calm while you ride the movement of it.

Wrap your leg once, way up high, then again around the calf. One wrap is also fine or you can put the toe on the floor.

Even though this leg looks straight here, in real life keep the standing leg as bent as possible.

Try to hold this pose for three to five breaths.

㉑ eagle pose

㉒ mountain pose

Let the softness of your front invite you to be open to whatever arises.

Bring your feet together and feel your weight dropping into the earth.

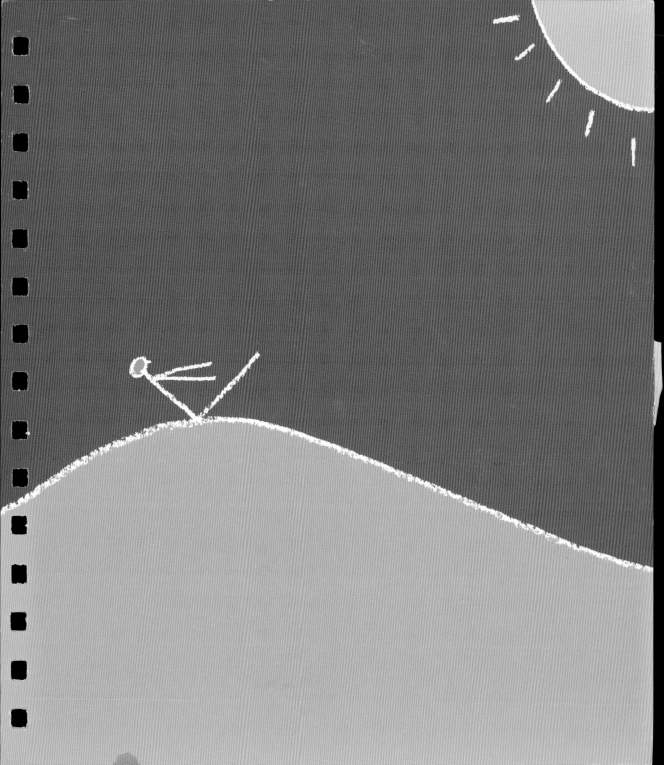

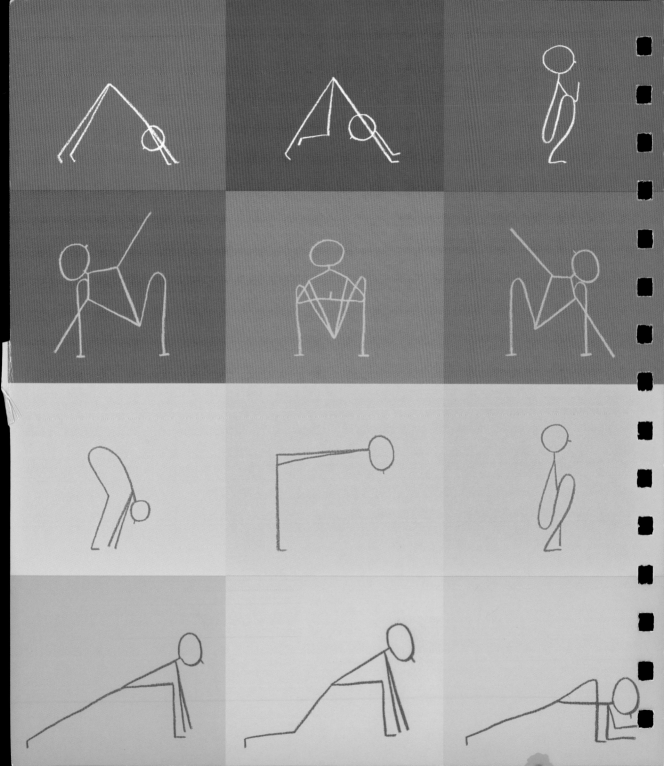

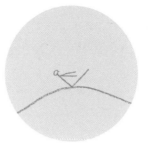

Thursday

Thursday is usually a tired day for my students. It's a good day to sit down and slow down. Seated poses rest the legs, calm the brain, and rejuvenate the entire system.

This series opens the hips, creating strength and stability for sitting meditation as well as increasing circulation to the pelvic region. The invigorating abdominal exercises also help strengthen the back and thighs. Through the squeezing and soaking effects of twisting, the internal organs get detoxified and then nourished. The forward bends are cooling and calming.

The fatigue that can arise on Thursday may be transformed through this seated-poses series. The total time for seated poses is seven minutes and five seconds. Hold each pose for five breaths or longer. Repeat #10–13 (lunging with hands inside foot, back knee down, forearms on the floor) to the second side before continuing with the rest of the sequence. Do #14 boat pose either three times for two breaths each, or once for five breaths—in and out. Do #17 side bend straddle stretch, #18 head to knee pose, and #19 rotated head to knee pose, to each side before continuing. Hold #20 for 3 breaths, unless it is too difficult—then instead repeat #14 boat pose. Be sure to do #22 twist to both sides.

Thursday's Practice: Seated Poses

1 downward dog

2 downward dog, walking feet to hands

3 squat with prayer hands

4 squat with side bend to the right

 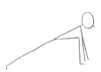 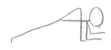

9 squat with hands inside feet

10 lunge with hands inside right foot

11 lunge with back leg bent

12 lunge with forearms on ground

   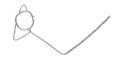

17 side bend straddle stretch

18 head to knee pose

19 rotated head to knee pose

20 half-boat pose

This sequence requires repeating from #10 through #13 with the left leg forward before continuing. Then do #14 through #16; repeat #17, #18, and #19 to both sides; do #20 and #21, repeat #22 to both sides; then end with #23.

5 squat with prayer hands

6 squat with side bend to the left

7 standing forward bend

8 standing forward bend with flat back and hands on thighs

13 squat with prayer hands

14 boat pose

15 cobbler's pose

16 straddle stretch

  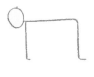

21 seated forward bend

22 twist

23 tabletop pose

Hold each pose for five breaths or longer. Repeat #10–#13 with the left leg in front before continuing with the rest of the sequence.

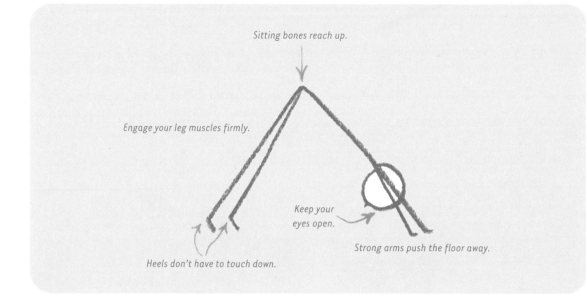

Sitting bones reach up.

Engage your leg muscles firmly.

Keep your eyes open.

Strong arms push the floor away.

Heels don't have to touch down.

① downward dog

③ squat with prayer hands

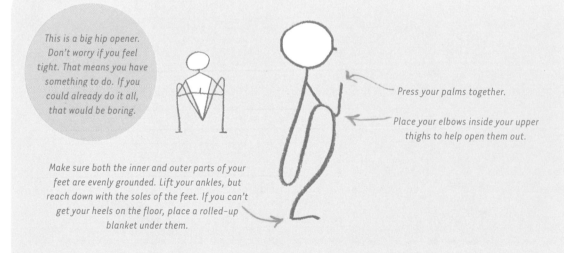

This is a big hip opener. Don't worry if you feel tight. That means you have something to do. If you could already do it all, that would be boring.

Press your palms together.

Place your elbows inside your upper thighs to help open them out.

Make sure both the inner and outer parts of your feet are evenly grounded. Lift your ankles, but reach down with the soles of the feet. If you can't get your heels on the floor, place a rolled-up blanket under them.

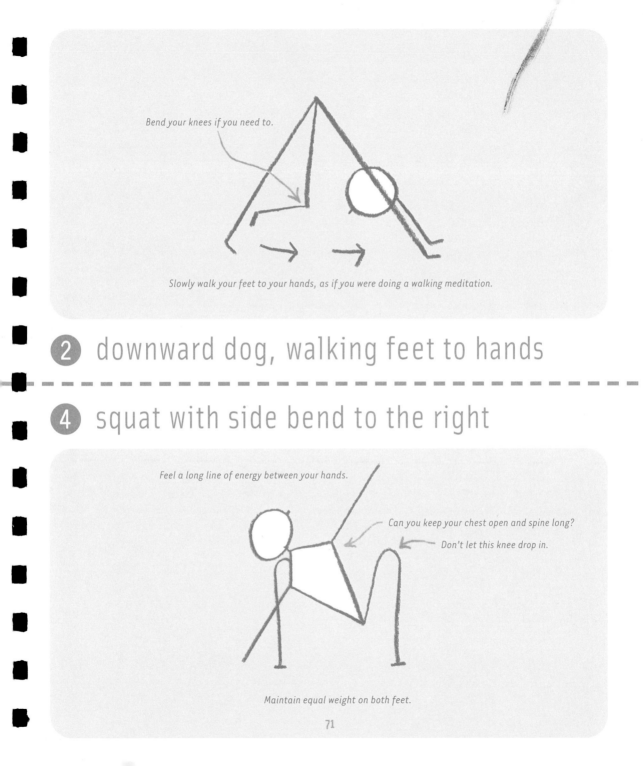

Bend your knees if you need to.

Slowly walk your feet to your hands, as if you were doing a walking meditation.

2 downward dog, walking feet to hands

4 squat with side bend to the right

Feel a long line of energy between your hands.

Can you keep your chest open and spine long?

Don't let this knee drop in.

Maintain equal weight on both feet.

71

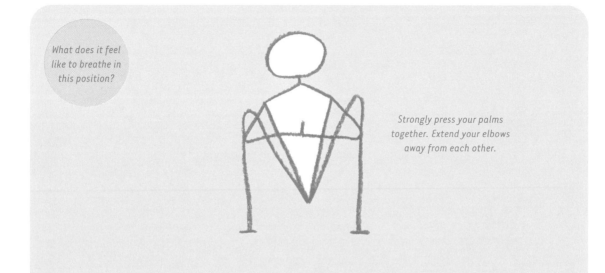

What does it feel like to breathe in this position?

Strongly press your palms together. Extend your elbows away from each other.

5 squat with prayer hands

7 standing forward bend

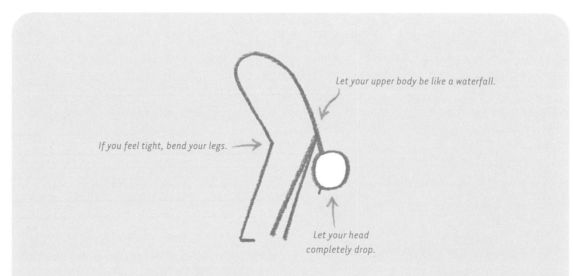

Let your upper body be like a waterfall.

If you feel tight, bend your legs. →

Let your head completely drop.

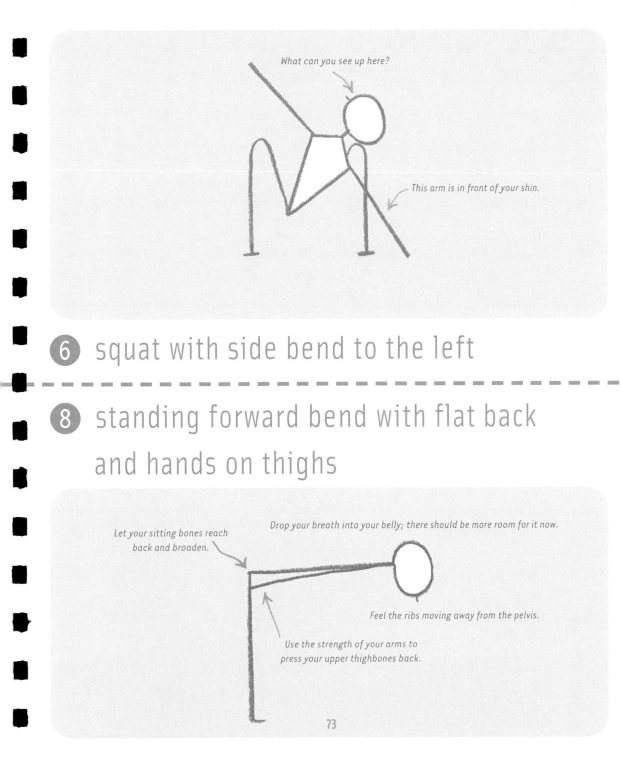

What can you see up here?

This arm is in front of your shin.

6 squat with side bend to the left

8 standing forward bend with flat back and hands on thighs

Let your sitting bones reach back and broaden.

Drop your breath into your belly; there should be more room for it now.

Feel the ribs moving away from the pelvis.

Use the strength of your arms to press your upper thighbones back.

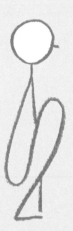

Try to touch the floor with your fingertips and still feel upright in your spine.

⑨ squat with hands inside feet

⑪ lunge with back leg bent

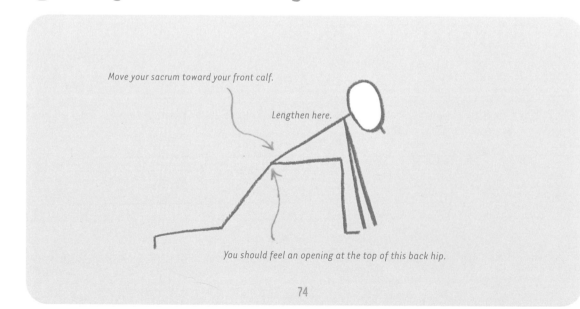

Move your sacrum toward your front calf.

Lengthen here.

You should feel an opening at the top of this back hip.

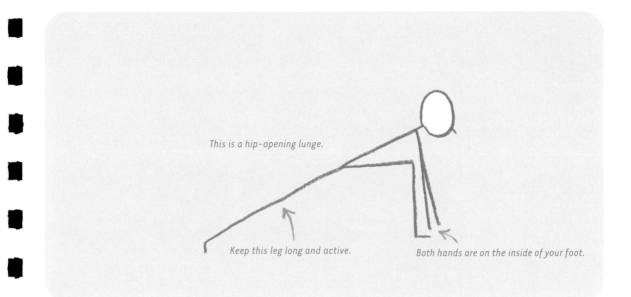

This is a hip-opening lunge.

Keep this leg long and active.

Both hands are on the inside of your foot.

⑩ lunge with hands inside right foot

⑫ lunge with forearms on ground

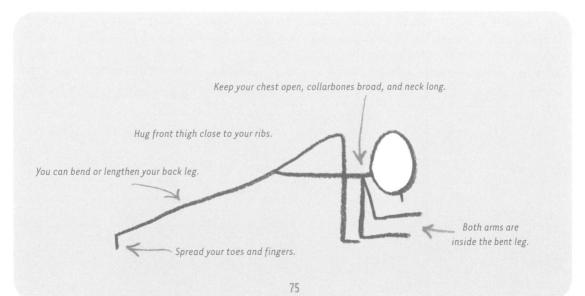

Keep your chest open, collarbones broad, and neck long.

Hug front thigh close to your ribs.

You can bend or lengthen your back leg.

Both arms are inside the bent leg.

Spread your toes and fingers.

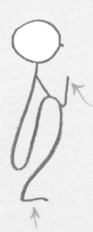

After you do this squat, repeat #10, #11, and #12, with the left leg forward. Step back into this squat and then continue this sequence.

Press your palms together.

Place your elbows inside your upper thighs to help open them out.

Make sure both the inner and outer parts of your feet are evenly grounded. Lift your ankles but reach down with the soles of the feet. If you can't get your heels on the floor, place a rolled-up blanket under them.

⑬ squat with prayer hands

⑮ cobbler's pose

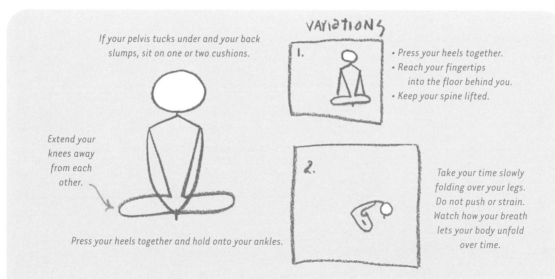

If your pelvis tucks under and your back slumps, sit on one or two cushions.

VARIATIONS

1.
• Press your heels together.
• Reach your fingertips into the floor behind you.
• Keep your spine lifted.

Extend your knees away from each other.

Press your heels together and hold onto your ankles.

2.
Take your time slowly folding over your legs. Do not push or strain. Watch how your breath lets your body unfold over time.

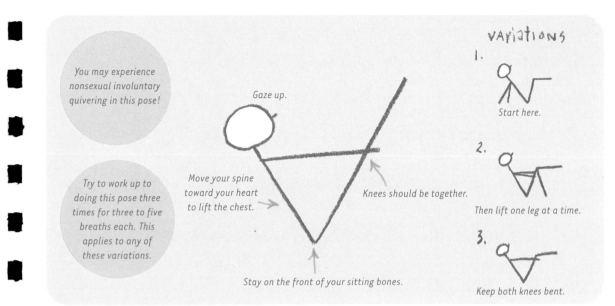

You may experience nonsexual involuntary quivering in this pose!

Try to work up to doing this pose three times for three to five breaths each. This applies to any of these variations.

Gaze up.

Move your spine toward your heart to lift the chest.

Knees should be together.

Stay on the front of your sitting bones.

vARiations

1.
Start here.

2.
Then lift one leg at a time.

3.
Keep both knees bent.

⑭ boat pose

- -

⑯ straddle stretch

Don't sacrifice the integrity of your alignment just to bend over.

You can use cushions under your sitting bones for this pose, too.

It takes quite a while for almost everybody to do this, so start here with your back straight, chest open, and fingertips on the floor slightly in front of you.

Eventually you may get your forearms down.

Keep your legs straight and active Extend your heels.

vAriations

1.

2.

Use a blanket or cushion.

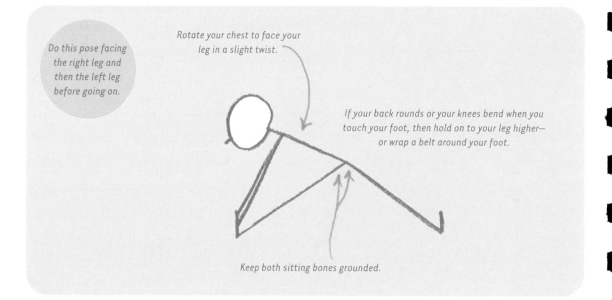

Do this pose facing the right leg and then the left leg before going on.

Rotate your chest to face your leg in a slight twist.

If your back rounds or your knees bend when you touch your foot, then hold on to your leg higher— or wrap a belt around your foot.

Keep both sitting bones grounded.

17 side bend straddle stretch

19 rotated head to knee pose

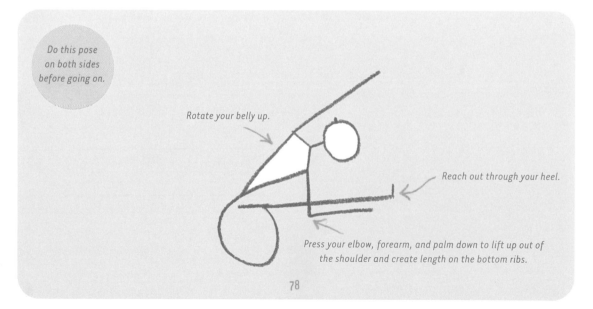

Do this pose on both sides before going on.

Rotate your belly up.

Reach out through your heel.

Press your elbow, forearm, and palm down to lift up out of the shoulder and create length on the bottom ribs.

Rotate your belly so that your
spine is centered over your leg.

Hold onto your foot, calf, thigh—wherever you can reach and
still maintain a long spine and open chest.

This leg is straight and active.

The sole of your foot is touching
the top of the inner thigh, like
in tree pose.

Do this pose facing
the right leg and
then the left leg
before going on.

⑱ head to knee pose

⑳ half-boat pose

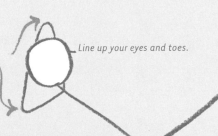

Try not to pull on your
neck but instead reach
the elbows away from
each other and rest your
head in your palms.

Line up your eyes and toes.

You may
experience nonsexual
involuntary quivering
during this pose, too!

Half-boat pose
is half again as hard as
regular boat. If it's too
much for you, do boat
pose or a beginner
variation again.

Lean toward the back of your sitting bones.

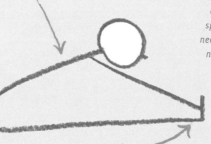

This pose is said to be calming. Is that your experience?

Make sure your chest is open and your breath is free. You never want your pose to inhibit your heart and lung activity.

Once again, hold on wherever you can reach and still keep your spine straight. Use a belt if you need to. Reach through your sternum, keeping the spine long as you fold over your legs.

Flex your feet.

㉑ seated-forward bend

- -

㉒ twist

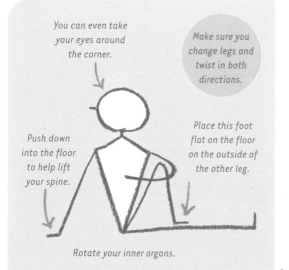

You can even take your eyes around the corner.

Make sure you change legs and twist in both directions.

Push down into the floor to help lift your spine.

Place this foot flat on the floor on the outside of the other leg.

Rotate your inner organs.

㉓ tabletop pose

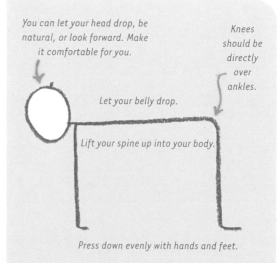

You can let your head drop, be natural, or look forward. Make it comfortable for you.

Knees should be directly over ankles.

Let your belly drop.

Lift your spine up into your body.

Press down evenly with hands and feet.

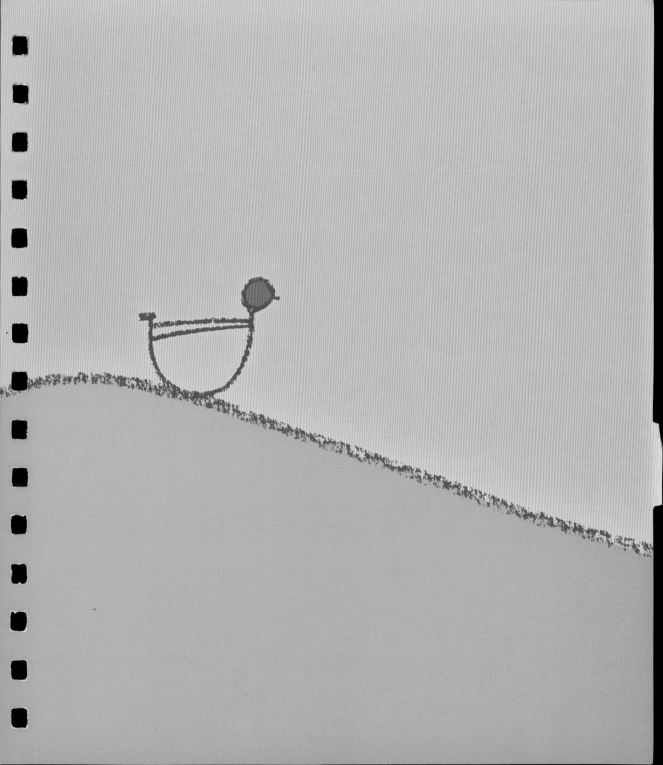

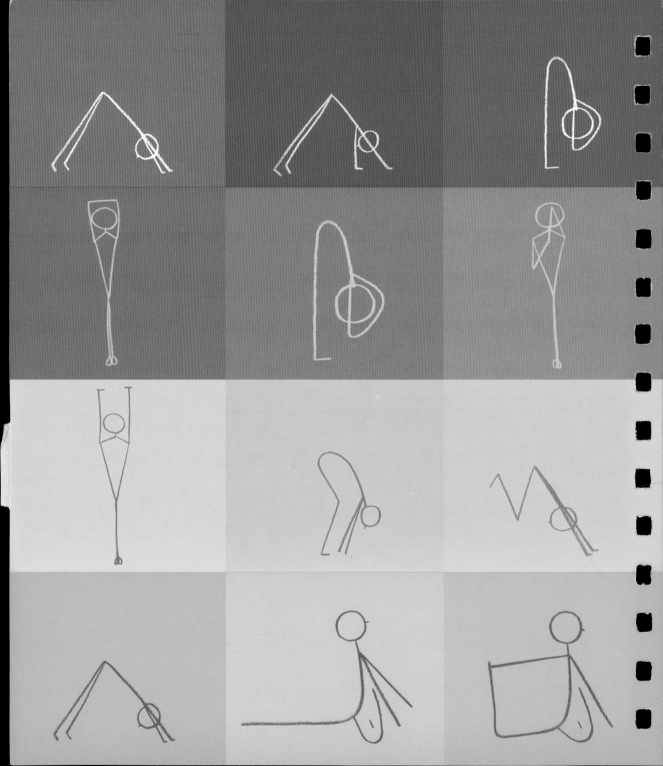

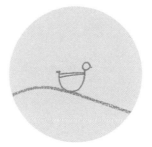

Friday

Just the fact that it's Friday can be enlivening, and can help you replace the weariness of Thursday with a sense of lightness and renewed vigor. And just in case that isn't your experience, back bends are a great way to cultivate joy, upbeat energy, and openheartedness.

Back bends increase flexibility in the spine; strengthen the back muscles; improve digestion; and open the heart, chest, and lungs.

Our daily activities such as driving or working at a computer invite us to round our shoulders, sink our chests, and generally slouch in our seats. This gets depressing. Back bends are an antidote to this pattern, encouraging us to get comfortable with feeling open in the front of our body. The vulnerability of that positioning in both the chest and the pelvis cultivates bravery and is actually rather thrilling. On an ordinary level, just relating to the fact that we have a back is the first step to sitting and standing tall.

The total time for back bending is ten minutes. Do #5 arm swings ten times on each arm. Make sure you do #6 shoulder stretch twice, changing arms. Try to work up to doing #16 bow pose three times.

Friday's Practice: Back Bending

1 downward dog

2 downward dog, walk hands to feet

3 standing forward bend, holding elbows

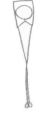

4 mountain pose holding elbows overhead

9 jump to downward dog

10 downward dog

11 pigeon pose

12 pigeon with thigh stretch

17 half-wheel

18 half-wheel with one leg up

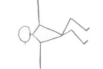

19 windshield wipers

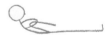

20 knee into chest

This sequence requires repeating #10 through #12, doing pigeon (#11 and #12) on the other side.

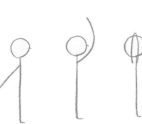 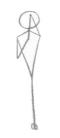 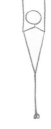

5 arm swings **6** shoulder stretch **7** mountain pose, arms up **8** standing forward bend

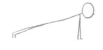 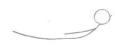

13 plank pose **14** knees, chest, chin **15** locust pose **16** bow pose

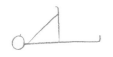

21 one leg up, laying on back **22** two legs up, laying on back **23** supine twist

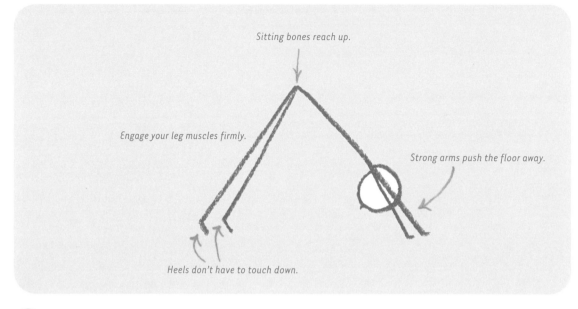

Sitting bones reach up.

Engage your leg muscles firmly.

Strong arms push the floor away.

Heels don't have to touch down.

1 downward dog

3 standing forward bend, holding elbows

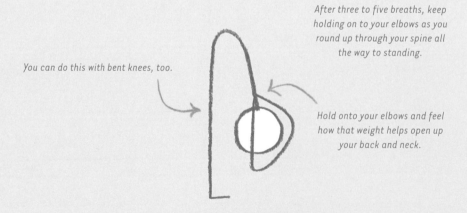

You can do this with bent knees, too.

After three to five breaths, keep holding on to your elbows as you round up through your spine all the way to standing.

Hold onto your elbows and feel how that weight helps open up your back and neck.

Let your weight drop down through your feet.

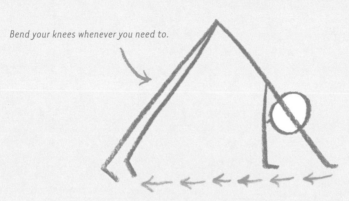

Bend your knees whenever you need to.

Slowly, hand by hand, walk yourself back to your feet.

2 downward dog, walk hands to feet

- -

4 mountain pose holding elbows overhead

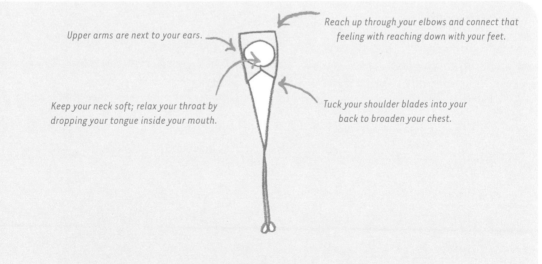

Upper arms are next to your ears.

Reach up through your elbows and connect that feeling with reaching down with your feet.

Keep your neck soft; relax your throat by dropping your tongue inside your mouth.

Tuck your shoulder blades into your back to broaden your chest.

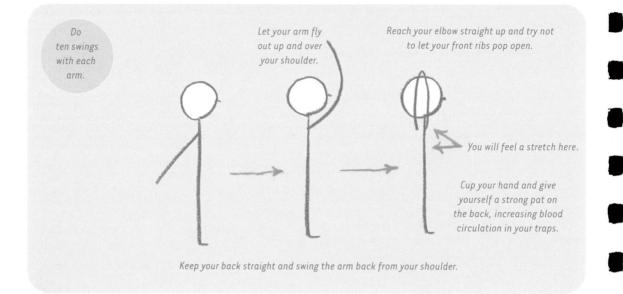

Do ten swings with each arm.

Let your arm fly out up and over your shoulder.

Reach your elbow straight up and try not to let your front ribs pop open.

You will feel a stretch here.

Cup your hand and give yourself a strong pat on the back, increasing blood circulation in your traps.

Keep your back straight and swing the arm back from your shoulder.

⑤ arm swings

⑦ mountain pose arms up

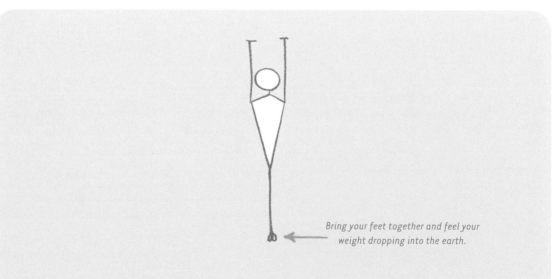

Bring your feet together and feel your weight dropping into the earth.

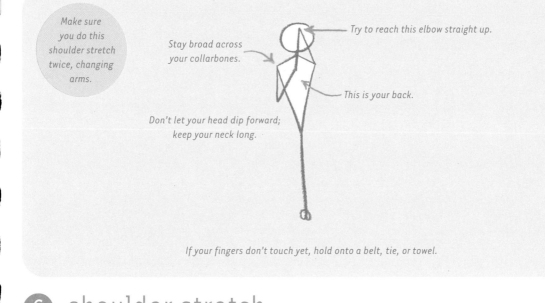

Make sure you do this shoulder stretch twice, changing arms.

Stay broad across your collarbones.

Try to reach this elbow straight up.

This is your back.

Don't let your head dip forward; keep your neck long.

If your fingers don't touch yet, hold onto a belt, tie, or towel.

6 shoulder stretch

8 standing forward bend

You can bend or straighten your legs.

Let your head completely drop.

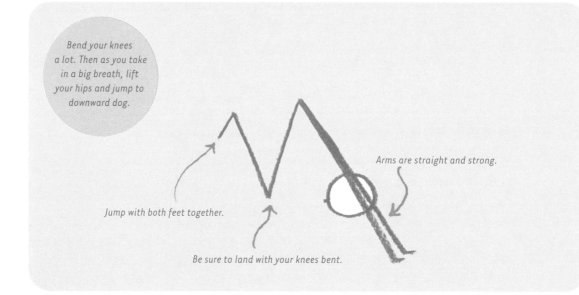

Bend your knees a lot. Then as you take in a big breath, lift your hips and jump to downward dog.

Arms are straight and strong.

Jump with both feet together.

Be sure to land with your knees bent.

⑨ jump to downward dog

⑪ pigeon pose

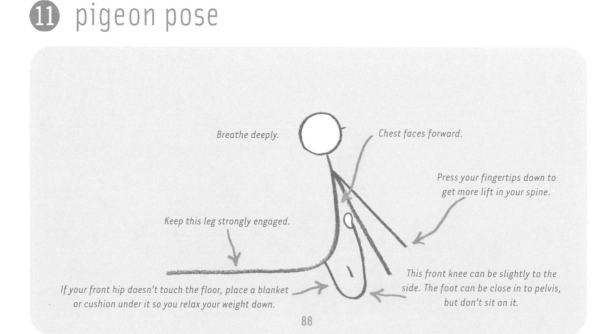

Breathe deeply.

Chest faces forward.

Press your fingertips down to get more lift in your spine.

Keep this leg strongly engaged.

If your front hip doesn't touch the floor, place a blanket or cushion under it so you relax your weight down.

This front knee can be slightly to the side. The foot can be close in to pelvis, but don't sit on it.

88

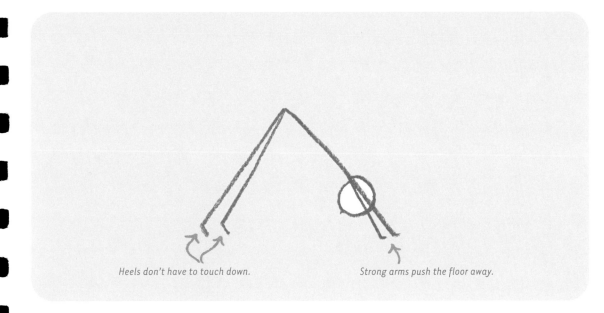

Heels don't have to touch down.

Strong arms push the floor away.

⑩ downward dog

⑫ pigeon with thigh stretch

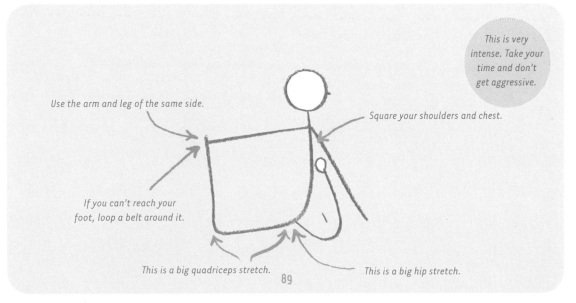

This is very intense. Take your time and don't get aggressive.

Use the arm and leg of the same side.

Square your shoulders and chest.

If you can't reach your foot, loop a belt around it.

This is a big quadriceps stretch.

This is a big hip stretch.

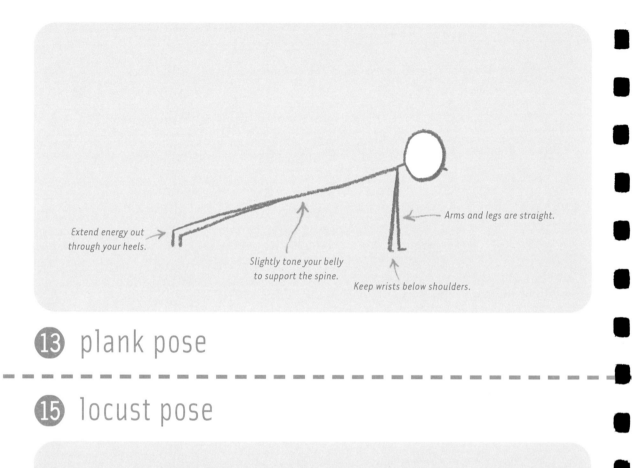

Extend energy out through your heels.

Slightly tone your belly to support the spine.

Arms and legs are straight.

Keep wrists below shoulders.

⑬ plank pose

⑮ locust pose

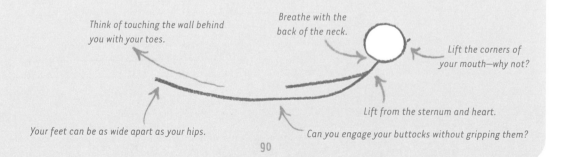

Think of touching the wall behind you with your toes.

Breathe with the back of the neck.

Lift the corners of your mouth—why not?

Lift from the sternum and heart.

Your feet can be as wide apart as your hips.

Can you engage your buttocks without gripping them?

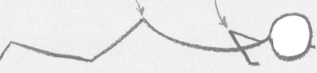

Sitting bones spin upward.

Keep your elbows tight into your ribs,
and palms flat on floor.

Lower your knees, chest, and chin to the floor.

⑭ knees chest chin

⑯ bow pose

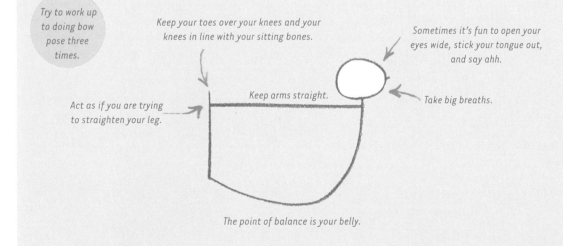

Try to work up
to doing bow
pose three
times.

Keep your toes over your knees and your
knees in line with your sitting bones.

Sometimes it's fun to open your
eyes wide, stick your tongue out,
and say ahh.

Act as if you are trying
to straighten your leg.

Keep arms straight.

Take big breaths.

The point of balance is your belly.

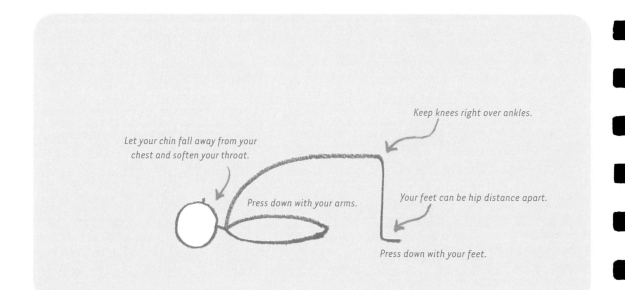

Keep knees right over ankles.

Let your chin fall away from your chest and soften your throat.

Press down with your arms.

Your feet can be hip distance apart.

Press down with your feet.

⑰ half-wheel

⑲ windshield wipers

Start with your feet flat on the floor slightly wider than your hips, then gently drop them to one side, then the other.

It's OK if this shoulder comes off the floor.

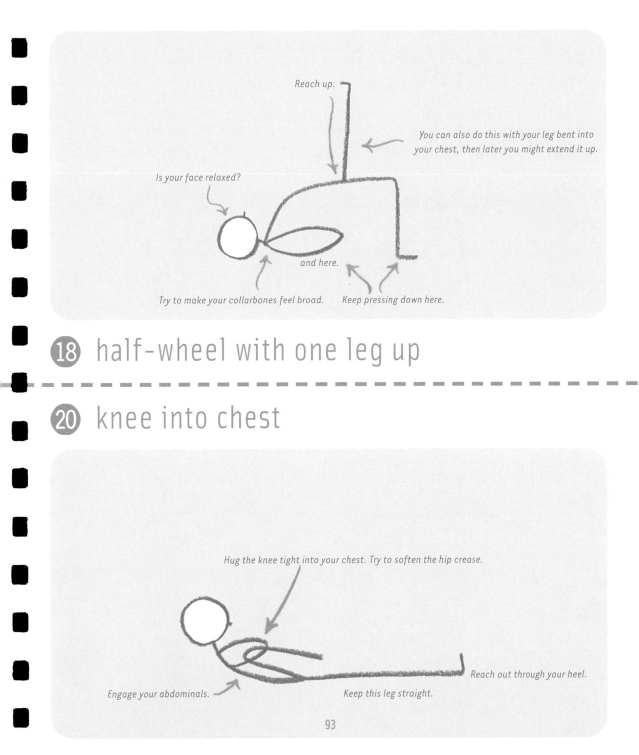

Reach up.

You can also do this with your leg bent into your chest, then later you might extend it up.

Is your face relaxed?

and here.

Try to make your collarbones feel broad. Keep pressing down here.

⑱ half-wheel with one leg up

⑳ knee into chest

Hug the knee tight into your chest. Try to soften the hip crease.

Reach out through your heel.

Engage your abdominals. Keep this leg straight.

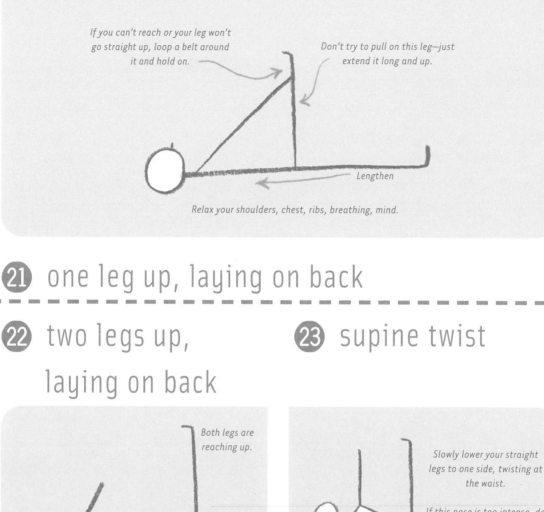

If you can't reach or your leg won't go straight up, loop a belt around it and hold on.

Don't try to pull on this leg—just extend it long and up.

Lengthen

Relax your shoulders, chest, ribs, breathing, mind.

21 one leg up, laying on back

22 two legs up, laying on back

Both legs are reaching up.

Activate your abdominals.

Press your palms down.

23 supine twist

Slowly lower your straight legs to one side, twisting at the waist.

If this pose is too intense, do it with your knees bent.

Press your palms and arms into the floor.

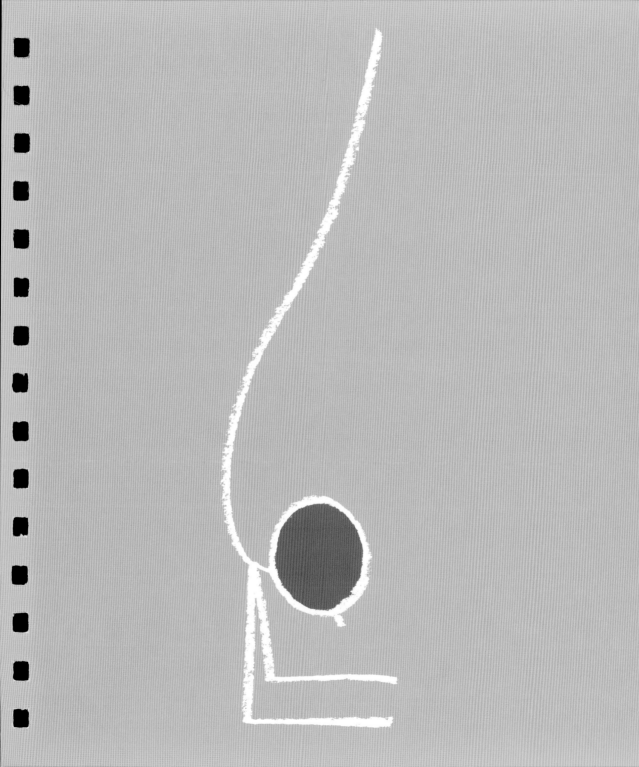

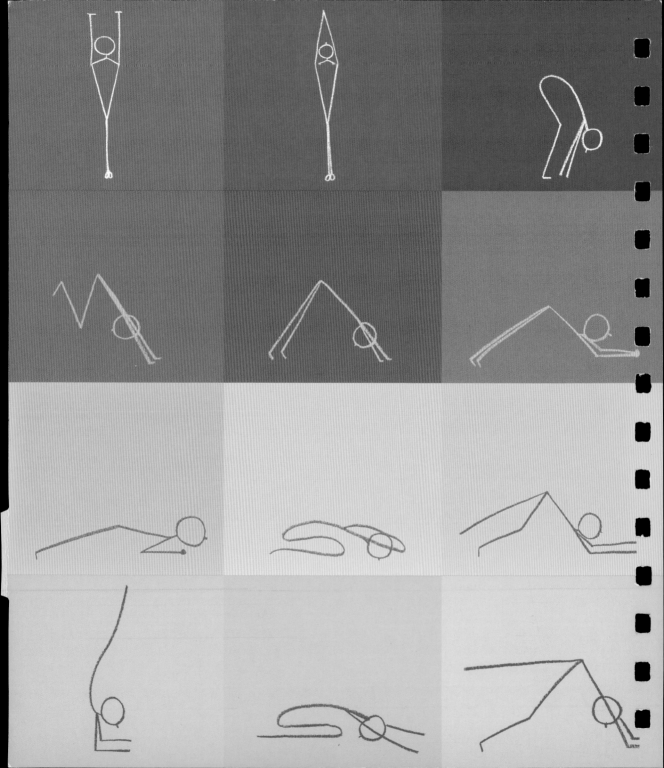

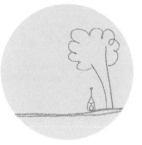

Saturday

Inversions give us a new perspective on our world. Turning upside down reminds us that nothing is solid, including our viewpoints, opinions, expectations, hopes, and fears. Since they are also a lot of fun, they are perfect to do on Saturday. It's not unusual to feel a little bit scared about doing inversions at first, so take your time and go step-by-step.

The king and queen of all asanas are inversions: the headstand, which generates heat, strengthens the arms and upper body, brings fresh blood to the brain, and activates the pituitary glands; and the shoulder stand, which has a cooling effect on the entire system, balances the thyroid, improves digestion, soothes the nerves, and relieves insomnia. So you can see that even though it may take time, it is worth it to learn how to invert. Once you do it, you will never be able to go back to a life without inverting.

Among the other benefits of inversions, the internal organs are massaged, the heart is strengthened, and the pull of gravity is reversed on the facial muscles and skin, giving a sort of natural face-lift.

It is recommended that menstruating women not do inversions during the first few days of their periods, so as not to interfere with the natural direction of the flow.

Saturday's Practice: Inversions

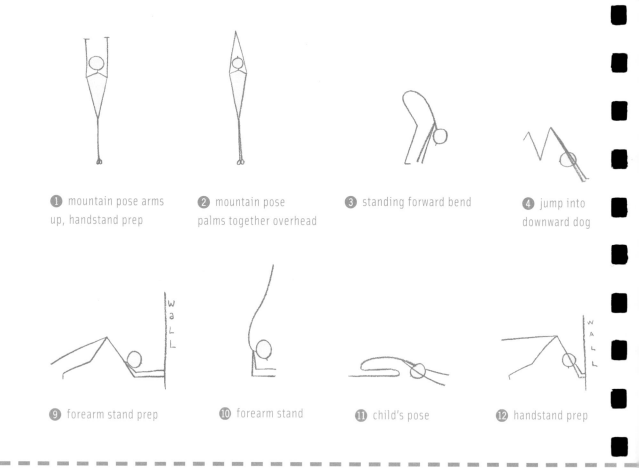

1 mountain pose arms up, handstand prep

2 mountain pose palms together overhead

3 standing forward bend

4 jump into downward dog

9 forearm stand prep

10 forearm stand

11 child's pose

12 handstand prep

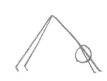 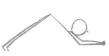 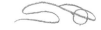 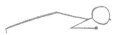

5 downward dog   **6** dolphin preparation   **7** dolphin   **8** child's pose with shoulder/tricep stretch

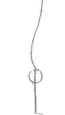 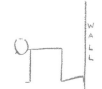 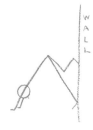

13 handstand   **14** l-shaped handstand prep   **15** l-shaped handstand walking up wall

*Take as much time as you need;
morning, afternoon, twilight,
Infinity . . . it's Saturday after all.*

Saturday's Practice: Inversions

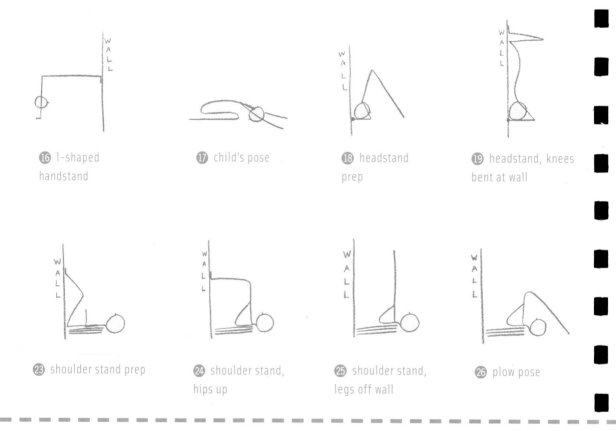

16 l-shaped handstand

17 child's pose

18 headstand prep

19 headstand, knees bent at wall

23 shoulder stand prep

24 shoulder stand, hips up

25 shoulder stand, legs off wall

26 plow pose

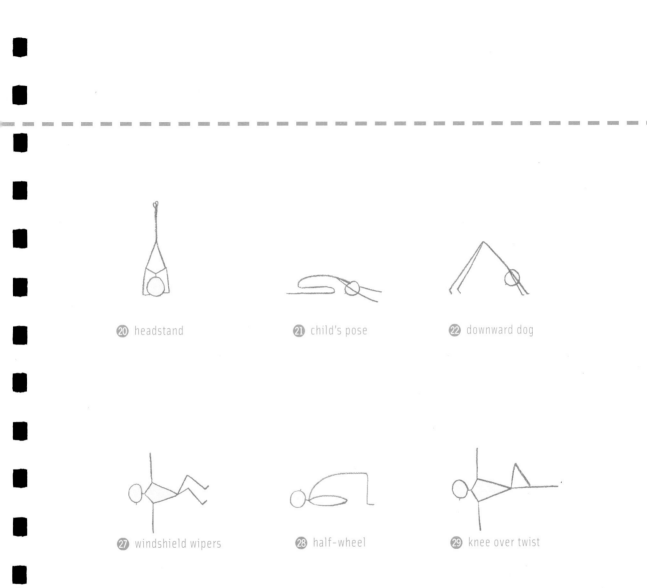

20 headstand

21 child's pose

22 downward dog

27 windshield wipers

28 half-wheel

29 knee over twist

Be sure to do the beginning of the sequence 1–8 and the end 27–29, but if you do not have time to do all the inversions, you can choose to work on just one (forearm stand, headstand, or shoulder stand) each time you do this practice.

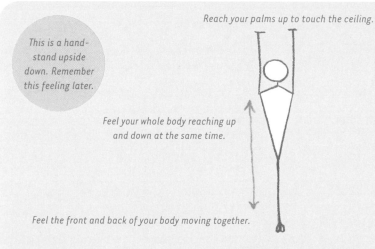

This is a hand-stand upside down. Remember this feeling later.

Reach your palms up to touch the ceiling.

Feel your whole body reaching up and down at the same time.

Feel the front and back of your body moving together.

Reach the soles of your feet down through the floor.

1 mountain pose arms up, handstand prep

3 standing forward bend

Let your upper body be like a waterfall pouring out of your strong legs.

Bend your knees if you are tight anywhere in back, including the back of your legs. If not, you can straighten your knees.

Let your head completely drop.

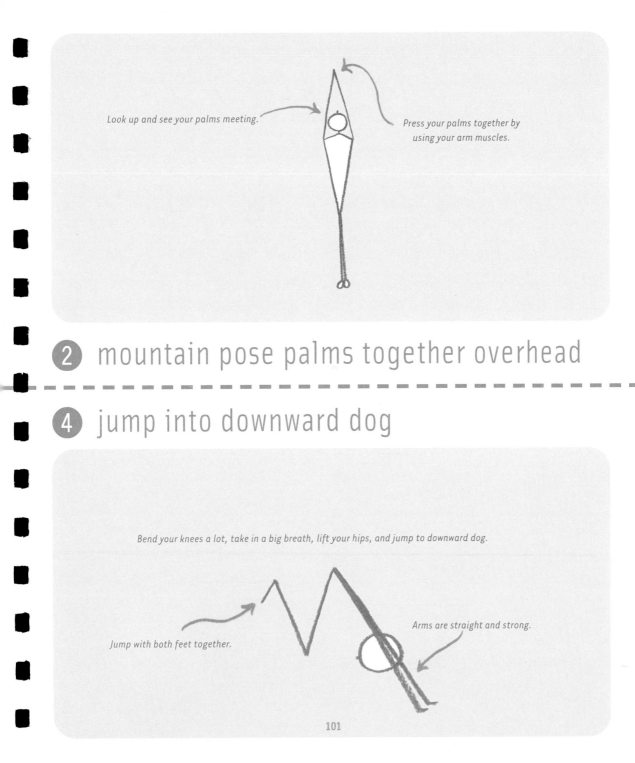

Look up and see your palms meeting.

Press your palms together by using your arm muscles.

2 mountain pose palms together overhead

4 jump into downward dog

Bend your knees a lot, take in a big breath, lift your hips, and jump to downward dog.

Jump with both feet together.

Arms are straight and strong.

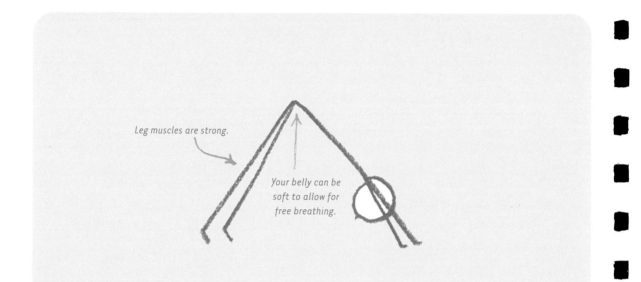

Leg muscles are strong.

Your belly can be soft to allow for free breathing.

5 downward dog

----

7 dolphin

One dolphin means going forward as you inhale and lifting the hips back up as you exhale.

Try not to collapse in your shoulders.

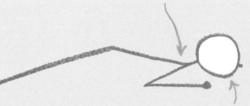

Lower your chin just past your hands.

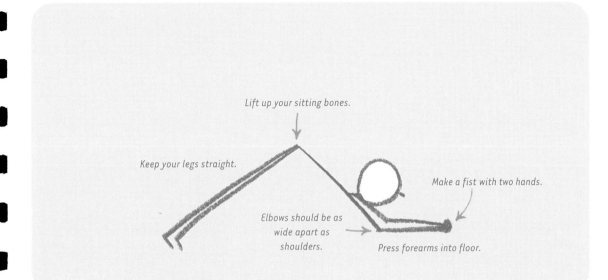

Lift up your sitting bones.

Keep your legs straight.

Make a fist with two hands.

Elbows should be as wide apart as shoulders.

Press forearms into floor.

6 dolphin preparation

8 child's pose with shoulder/tricep stretch

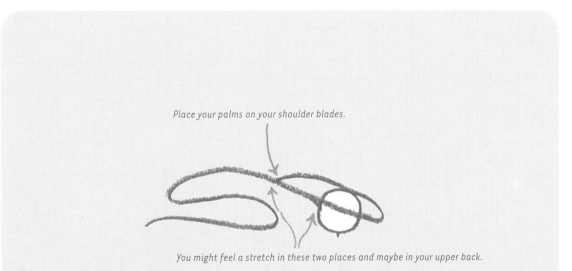

Place your palms on your shoulder blades.

You might feel a stretch in these two places and maybe in your upper back.

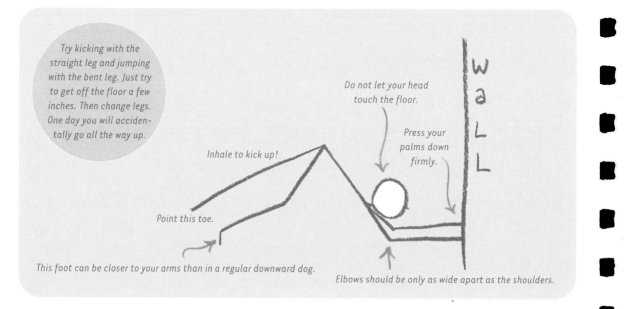

Try kicking with the straight leg and jumping with the bent leg. Just try to get off the floor a few inches. Then change legs. One day you will accidentally go all the way up.

Inhale to kick up!

Do not let your head touch the floor.

Press your palms down firmly.

W a L L

Point this toe.

This foot can be closer to your arms than in a regular downward dog.

Elbows should be only as wide apart as the shoulders.

⑨ forearm stand prep

⑪ child's pose

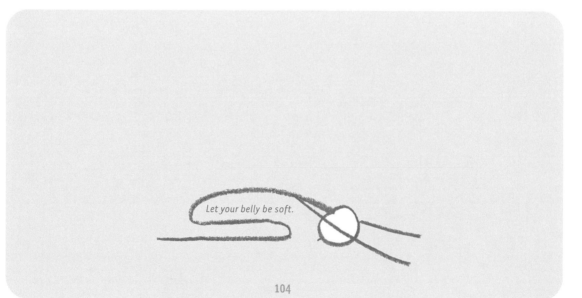

Let your belly be soft.

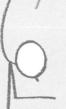

Try to stay up here for three to five breaths. Don't forget to breathe!

Reach up strongly with your tailbone, send energy up through inner thighs and inner heels.

Soften your front ribs and feel your breath in your back.

Keep your palms flat and in line with your elbows and shoulders.

⑩ forearm stand

- -

⑫ handstand prep

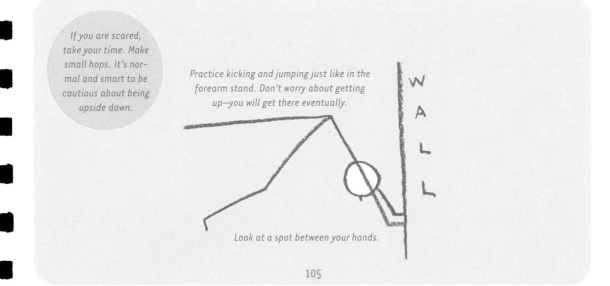

If you are scared, take your time. Make small hops. It's normal and smart to be cautious about being upside down.

Practice kicking and jumping just like in the forearm stand. Don't worry about getting up—you will get there eventually.

W
A
L
L

Look at a spot between your hands.

Try to work up to standing on your hands for three to five breaths.

Extend through the balls of your feet. Keep a sense of space in your ankles. (Have Barbie doll feet.)

Practice this at the wall. To balance, place your feet on the wall with your fingertips about six inches from the wall. Squeeze your thighs together and keep your arms straight by pushing down.

⑬ handstand

⑮ l-shaped handstand walking up wall

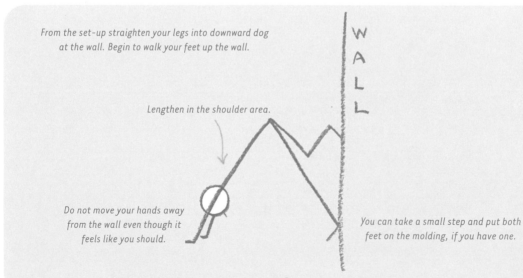

From the set-up straighten your legs into downward dog at the wall. Begin to walk your feet up the wall.

Lengthen in the shoulder area.

W
A
L
L

Do not move your hands away from the wall even though it feels like you should.

You can take a small step and put both feet on the molding, if you have one.

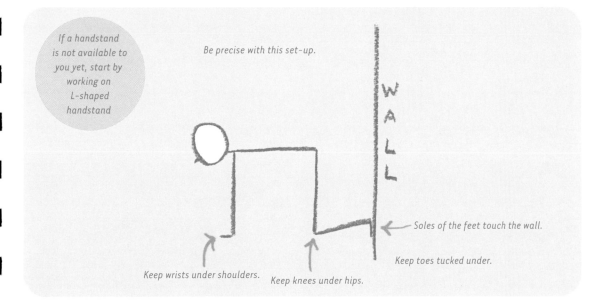

If a handstand is not available to you yet, start by working on L-shaped handstand

Be precise with this set-up.

WALL

Soles of the feet touch the wall.

Keep toes tucked under.

Keep wrists under shoulders.

Keep knees under hips.

14 L-shaped handstand prep

16 L-shaped handstand

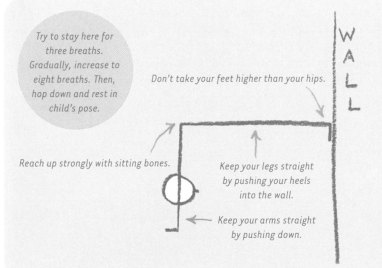

Try to stay here for three breaths. Gradually, increase to eight breaths. Then, hop down and rest in child's pose.

Don't take your feet higher than your hips.

WALL

Reach up strongly with sitting bones.

Keep your legs straight by pushing your heels into the wall.

Keep your arms straight by pushing down.

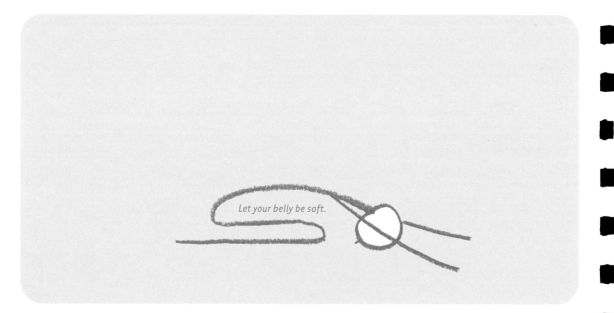

Let your belly be soft.

⑰ child's pose

---

⑲ headstand, knees bent at wall

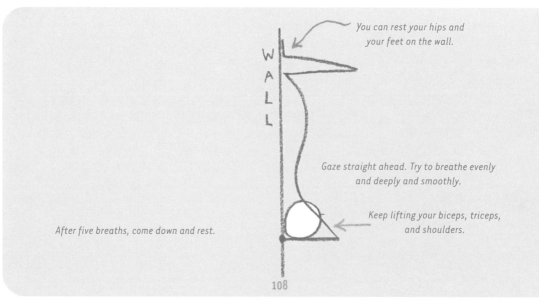

You can rest your hips and your feet on the wall.

W
A
L
L

Gaze straight ahead. Try to breathe evenly and deeply and smoothly.

Keep lifting your biceps, triceps, and shoulders.

After five breaths, come down and rest.

Interlace your fingers and make a fist. Elbows should be as wide apart as shoulders—no wider. Place the top of your head on the floor, right behind your fist. Do not put your head in your hands.

VARIATIONS

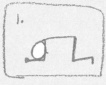

1.

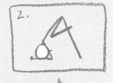

2.

W
A
L
L

Keep lifting up here.

Keep your neck long.

Start like this to get used to feeling your head on the floor. →

Make sure you are using your arm strength here so not all your weight is on your head.

Reach your shoulders up toward your waist.

Eventually you can straighten one leg with the other knee bent into your chest.

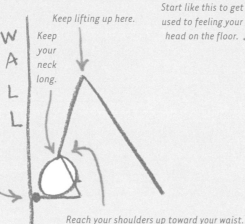

⑱ headstand prep

⑳ headstand

Draw your legs together and extend up through your toes and heels.

Move front ribs and waist into your back.

Press down with forearms, up with upper arms.

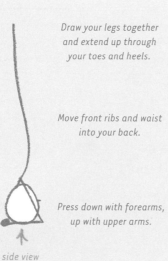

side view

The headstand is one of the most beneficial poses in yoga. But it takes a lot of strength and confidence. Take it one step at a time.

Very slowly, over a period of many weeks or even months or years, try to work up to a ten-breath-long headstand.

front view

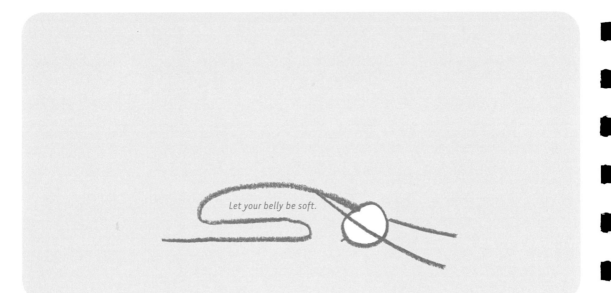

Let your belly be soft.

21 child's pose

23 shoulder stand prep

WALL

When you get organized into this set-up, press your elbows down at the same time that you push your feet into the wall, and your hips will go right up.

Fold up three firm blankets and place them under your back.

Your neck and head should not be touching the blanket.

110

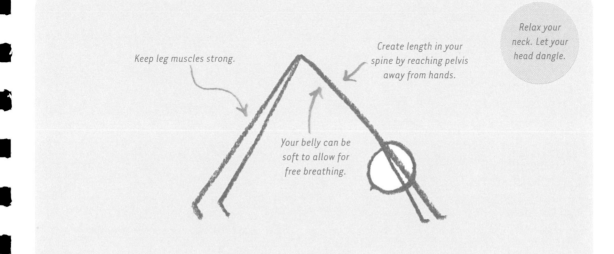

Keep leg muscles strong.

Create length in your spine by reaching pelvis away from hands.

Relax your neck. Let your head dangle.

Your belly can be soft to allow for free breathing.

㉒ downward dog

㉔ shoulder stand, hips up

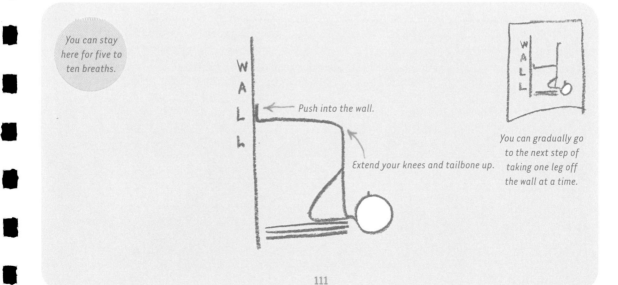

You can stay here for five to ten breaths.

Push into the wall.

Extend your knees and tailbone up.

You can gradually go to the next step of taking one leg off the wall at a time.

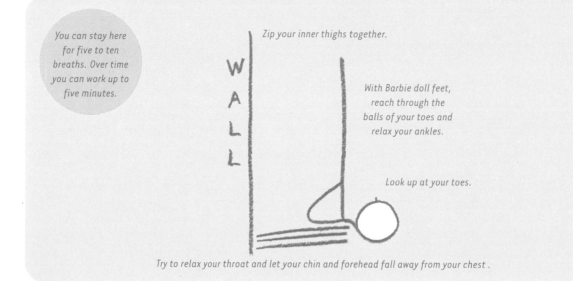

You can stay here for five to ten breaths. Over time you can work up to five minutes.

Zip your inner thighs together.

W
A
L
L

With Barbie doll feet, reach through the balls of your toes and relax your ankles.

Look up at your toes.

Try to relax your throat and let your chin and forehead fall away from your chest .

25 shoulder stand, legs off wall

27 windshield wipers

Start with your feet flat on the floor slightly wider than your hips, then gently drop them to one side, then the other.

It's OK if this shoulder comes off the floor.

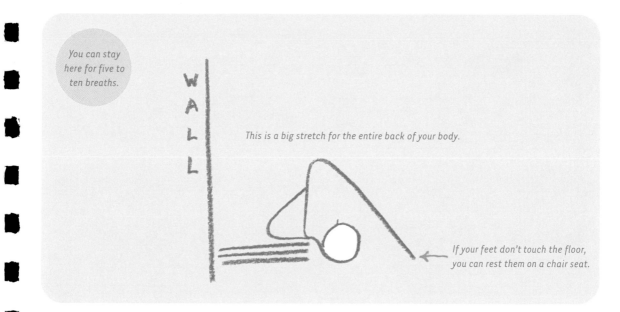

You can stay here for five to ten breaths.

WALL

This is a big stretch for the entire back of your body.

If your feet don't touch the floor, you can rest them on a chair seat.

26 plow pose

28 half-wheel

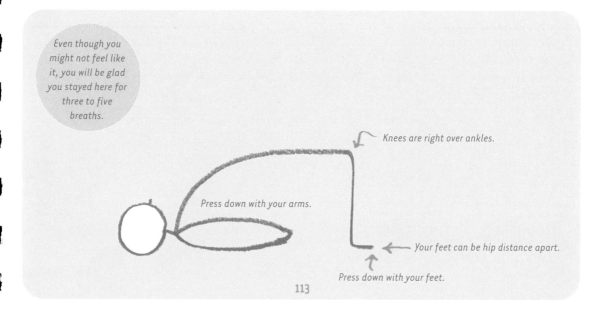

Even though you might not feel like it, you will be glad you stayed here for three to five breaths.

Knees are right over ankles.

Press down with your arms.

Your feet can be hip distance apart.

Press down with your feet.

113

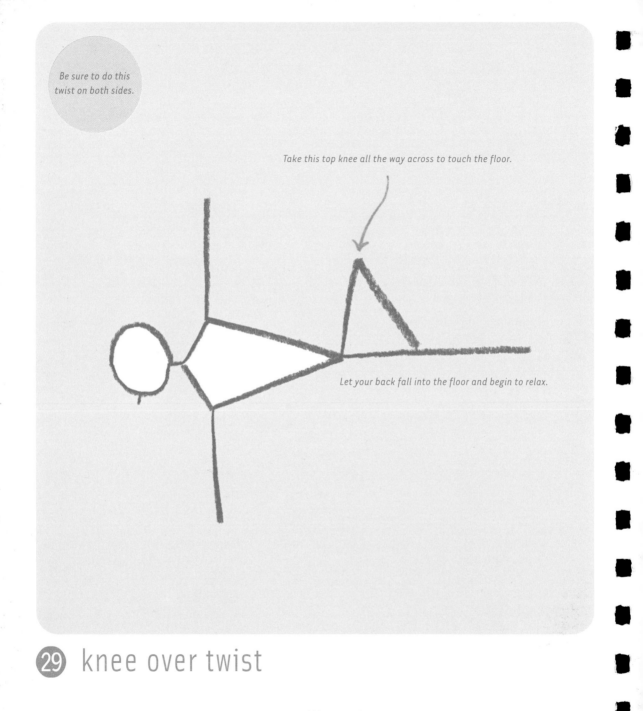

Be sure to do this twist on both sides.

Take this top knee all the way across to touch the floor.

Let your back fall into the floor and begin to relax.

29 knee over twist

114

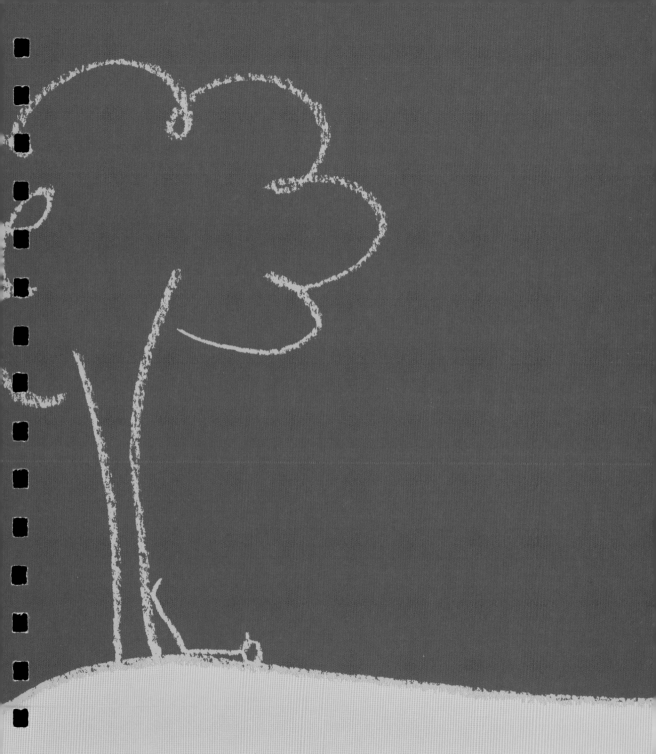

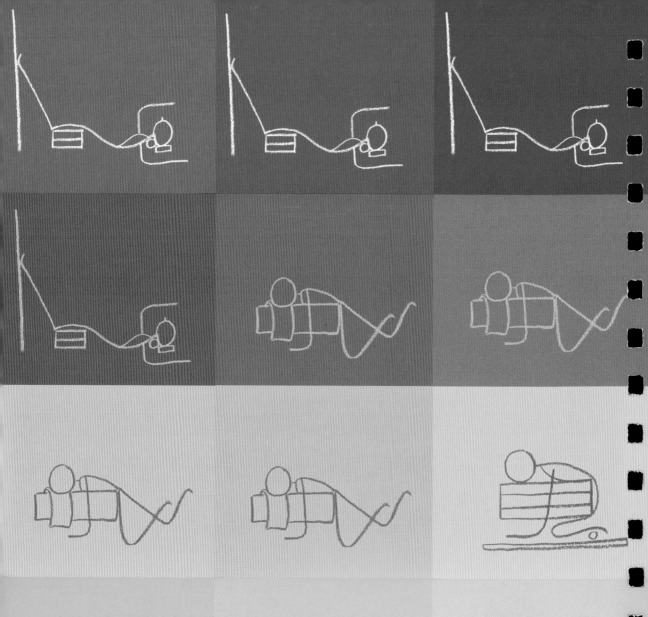

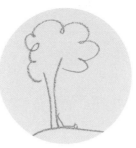

Sunday

Relaxation is considered one of the most important aspects of yoga and completely unique to this method of body/mind training. Instead of us doing yoga, this is the time when yoga does us. Our only job is to receive the benefits of the practice. This is a good lesson for many of us. We don't have to be active for something to happen.

Our body holds tension in our muscles, and we're not even aware of it. Restorative yoga is a way to gain this awareness without judgment or concern and to practice letting go of physical contraction, which is closely aligned with mental and emotional contraction. If we can be open and observant, we will begin to notice our body releasing and opening on its own, little by little, breath by breath.

It's a good idea to do a weekly restorative yoga practice, and Sunday is the perfect day for it. If you think of Sunday as the beginning of the week, this will give you a sense of spaciousness and receptivity to whatever may arise during your week. If you think of Sunday as the end of a busy week, restorative postures will help you assimilate your experiences and feel refreshed for what comes next.

You can do this sequence of restorative postures as your entire yoga session for the day. Begin with sitting and breathing, go right to restorative practice, and finish with the daily relaxation. (If you want to start with something a little active, you can still do the daily warm-up first.) If you have time, this would be a good day to extend your sitting meditation period to at least twenty minutes.

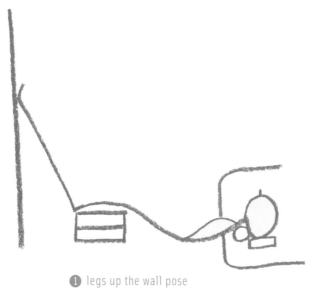

1 legs up the wall pose

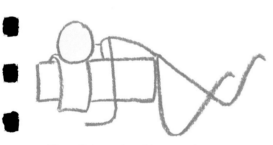

2 reclining twist with support

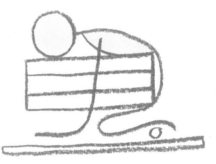

3 supported child's pose

You can stay in each pose as long as you want. Try to stay at least fifteen to twenty minutes in each.

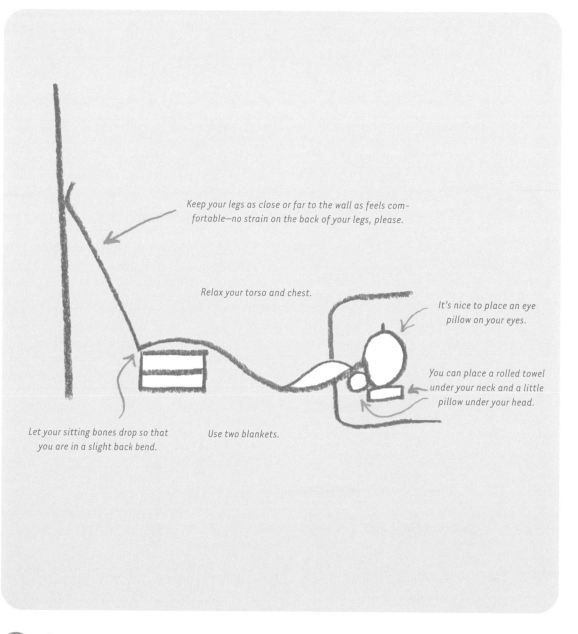

Keep your legs as close or far to the wall as feels comfortable—no strain on the back of your legs, please.

Relax your torso and chest.

It's nice to place an eye pillow on your eyes.

You can place a rolled towel under your neck and a little pillow under your head.

Let your sitting bones drop so that you are in a slight back bend.

Use two blankets.

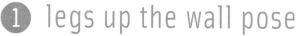 **legs up the wall pose**

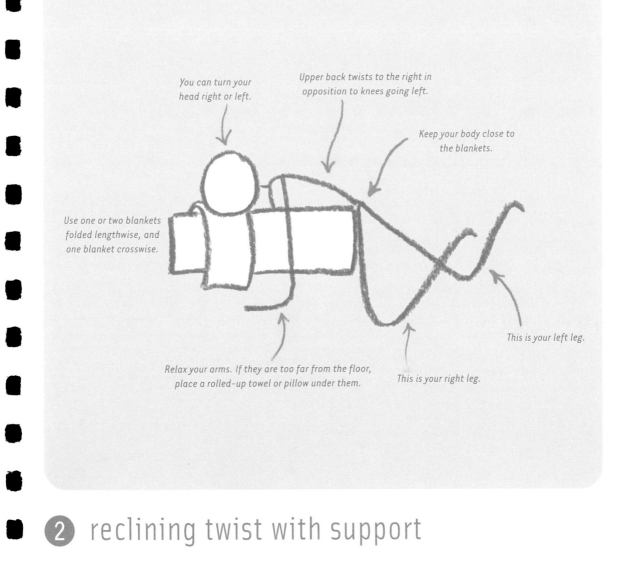

You can turn your head right or left.

Upper back twists to the right in opposition to knees going left.

Keep your body close to the blankets.

Use one or two blankets folded lengthwise, and one blanket crosswise.

This is your left leg.

Relax your arms. If they are too far from the floor, place a rolled-up towel or pillow under them.

This is your right leg.

② reclining twist with support

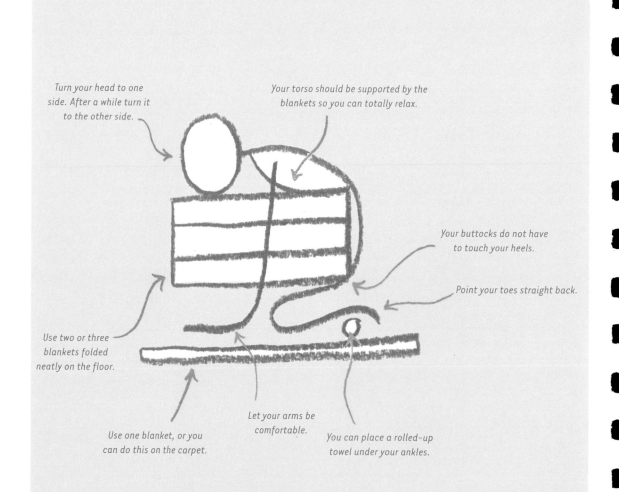

Turn your head to one side. After a while turn it to the other side.

Your torso should be supported by the blankets so you can totally relax.

Your buttocks do not have to touch your heels.

Point your toes straight back.

Use two or three blankets folded neatly on the floor.

Use one blanket, or you can do this on the carpet.

Let your arms be comfortable.

You can place a rolled-up towel under your ankles.

③ supported child's pose

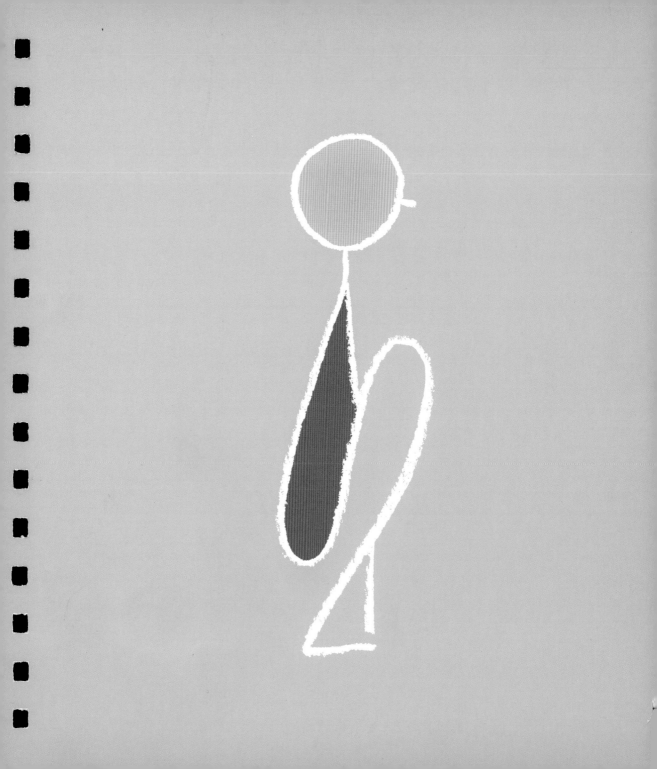

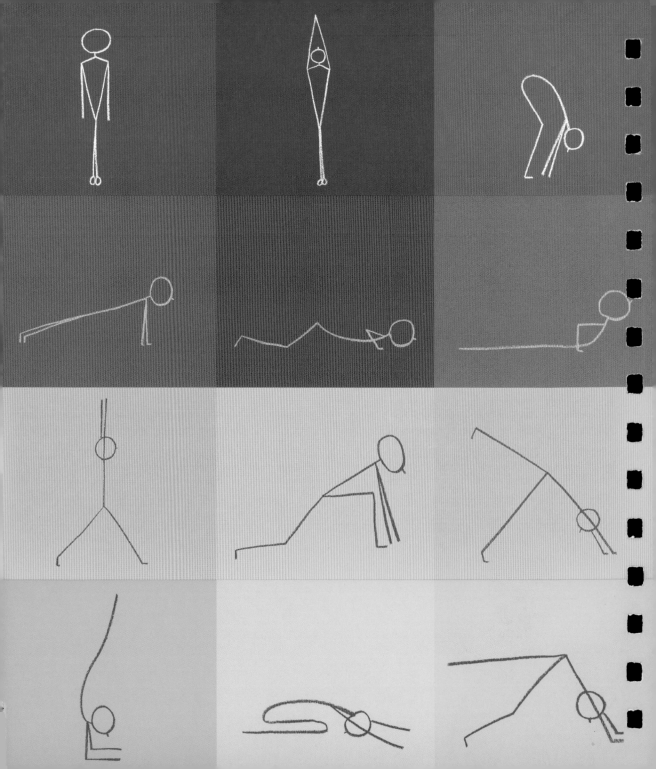

Recipes: How to Put It All Together

The following recipes are combinations of yoga postures that make a complete practice appropriate for various situations. Choose one and then go through the book, marking the pages that illustrate the poses you will be doing for the day's recipe. It's important that you do the poses in the order given. You can explore for yourself any transitional movements that you have learned from the daily practice sessions or create some of your own.

•Brand-New Beginners

Daily warm-up; Monday #1, 2, 3, 2, 1, tree pose, corpse pose

•Thirty-Minute Practice

Daily warm-up; sun salute two times on each side; standing poses #1–7, warrior two, circle arms to downward dog; child's pose, cobbler's pose, head to knee, seated forward bend, seated twist, half-wheel three times for five breaths each, windshield wipers, shoulder stand, corpse pose

•One-Hour Practice

Daily warm-up two times, sun salute three times each side, all standing poses, all balancing poses, all seated poses, headstand, handstand or forearm stand, all back bending poses, corpse pose

•Strength Practice

Daily warm-up, sun salute three times on each side, all the balancing poses, boat pose three times for five breaths each, half-boat, dolphin (five), forearm stand, l-shaped hand-stand, half-wheel, half-wheel with one leg up, laying on back with two legs up into supine twist, shoulder stand, plow pose, corpse pose

•Morning Practice

Daily warm-up, sun salute two times, headstand or prep, back bending #1–14 both sides, locust, bow, windshield wipers, shoulder stand, plow, corpse pose

•Before Bedtime

Daily warm-up, cobbler's pose, straddle stretch, side bend straddle, head to knee pose, rotated head to knee pose, legs up the wall, corpse pose

Sitting Meditation

Mindfulness meditation technique helps us begin to notice when we are spacing out, doing things by habit and not by choice. It gives us a sense of how everything keeps changing and how it is possible to stay composed within life's ups and downs. It doesn't take us away to a land of bliss but instead opens us up to our immediate experiences, which include moments of bliss as well as frustrations, hurt, confusion, and joy.

Meditative awareness is what distinguishes yoga practice from other forms of physical fitness. It is what helps us connect what we experience in our yoga practice with the rest of our life. Here's how you do it:

- Take your seat on a firm pillow or cushion.
- Place your palms on your thighs in the mudra of calm abiding.
- Open your eyes about halfway and let your gaze rest on the floor about four or five feet in front of you. Let your eyes relax, without getting fuzzy.
- Place your attention on your breathing. Let your breath go in and out naturally. Whenever you notice that you are thinking, which will happen a lot, gently say to yourself, "thinking," and return your attention to your breath.

Mindfulness meditation is not about emptying your brain. It is a method for becoming aware of the habits of your mind, letting go of your thoughts when you notice them, and once again resting in the present moment. This is a traditional Tibetan Buddhist meditation technique called *shamatha,* or calm abiding.

You may also begin to experience discomfort—aching back, whining hips, sleeping legs. It is fine to shift your posture if your physical pain becomes too much. When you move, you still follow the technique of watching the breath and labeling, "thinking." Make sure that when you move it is because you really need to and not because you are bored and restless.

Pictured on the facing page are three recommended ways to move in meditation:

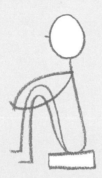

if your hips and knees hurt

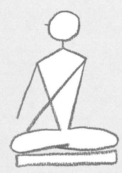

if your back and neck hurt

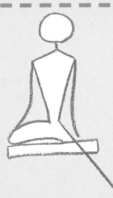

if your leg falls asleep

123

Walking Meditation

Walking meditation is a way to begin to take your mindfulness into your everyday world. It is a transitional practice between watching your mind while sitting still and maintaining your awareness while interacting with places, people, and things. The world will look more vivid and brighter than usual when you do this practice—like seeing things for the first time.

Try walking slowly down the street for one block. You don't have to go in slow motion, but take your pace down several notches from how you walk when you want to get somewhere. Keep your steps steady and even.

In sitting meditation we use the breath as a reference point for returning to and resting in the present moment, but in walking meditation you use your footsteps. Try to stay present with every footfall—heel, ball, toe. When you realize you've spaced out and gotten caught up in a thought, it's no big deal. Simply return your mind to the experience of walking.

Rest your gaze at eye level and include things in your peripheral vision. Extend your awareness to your environment as you move through your world. Feel your feet connecting to the earth. Hear the sounds around you. Smell and taste whatever comes your way. Let your thoughts come and go.

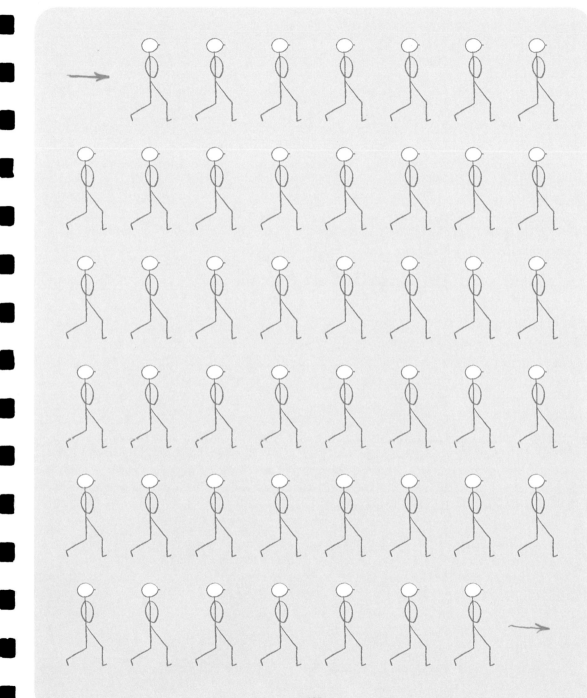

Glossary

Asana: This word refers to the physical postures of hatha yoga practice. It means "seat" or the part of your body that is touching the ground. For example, with the word *sirsasana*, *sirsa* is "head," and asana means "seat" so it means put your head on the ground or headstand.

Breathing: Conscious manipulated breathing is an essential part of yoga and traditionally called *pranayama. Prana* means "life force" and can be found in air, water, earth, sunshine, and humans, and animals. We can most easily experience it and control it through conscious manipulated breathing techniques. *Ayama* means "extension," so *pranayama* is a series of breathing exercises designed to lengthen life as well as to improve the quality of it. Yogis say that each person has a predetermined number of breaths for their life, so the theory is that if you can learn to lengthen each breath, you will live longer.

Hatha: This often translates as "forceful" and refers to the energy and effort that is involved in asana practice. We often think of yoga as relaxing, but it takes strength of mind as well as muscle to hold your body in an asana for more than two seconds. This effort is part of the path to discovering spaciousness. Hatha yoga teaches us that rather than being aggressive, willpower can mean being wakeful, focused, and on the dot. This balance is also implied in the word *hatha. Ha* means "sun," which yoga philosophy considers to have masculine qualities of activity, heat, outward energy, and light. *Tha* means moon, which contains the feminine qualities of receptivity, coolness, turning inward, and darkness.

Mudra: A physical seal, such as placing the thumb and first finger together, which creates a specific energetic circuit that will create a certain experience. For example, placing your palms flat on your thighs is called the mudra of calm abiding. You may feel that turning your palms down is like gently putting a lid on your overstimulated nervous system.

If you are sleepy while meditating, it is recommended that you use the cosmic mudra, which is palms turned up, fingers of one hand on top of the other with your thumb tips lightly touching. This mudra should be held slightly above your lap, and if you start to fall asleep your hands will drop and awaken you.

Some asanas, such as the shoulder stand, are also considered mudras.

Om: The sound of Om is created from four parts: A, U, M, and the silence after the sound. The silence is called the *turiya* and is said to include all the sounds of the universe. It can be felt as a vibration and reminds us that all the sounds we hear—our heartbeats, thunder, birds singing, even jackhammers—are all sound manifestations of the pulsation of the cosmos that moves through all of us all the time.

Prana: Life force or primordial energy that flows through all living beings. *Prana* can also be found in elements that create life, such as sunlight, water, and earth.

Savasana: This is one of the most important poses in yoga practice. It is translated as the corpse pose and is traditionally done at the end of every yoga class. It gives our bodies a chance to assimilate all the benefits of the more active poses, as well as a chance for our body temperature to cool down after vigorous practice. Although it seems that *savasana* is like taking a nap, it has the same dynamic as all yoga poses, which is a balance of wakefulness and relaxation. So although your body may be still, in *savasana* yogis are invited to watch their minds and remain alert, just as in meditation practice.

Shamatha: Traditional Tibetan Buddhist meditation technique that means "calm abiding" or "resting in peace." It is done with the eyes open, using the breath as a reference point for returning to and resting in the present moment. This method of one-pointed concentration leads to an increased ability to concentrate and is the ground for yoga practice and more advanced meditation techniques.

In walking meditation, *shamatha* is merged with *vipassana*, or a lifting of the eyes during which the meditator begins to experience a larger awareness of the environment in her consciousness.

Vinyasa: This refers to a flowing form of yoga in which asanas are strung together like beads on a necklace, and the string that connects them is the breath. It can be done slowly and spaciously or faster, giving each asana only one breath. This form generates heat, cultivates coordination and gracefulness, and reminds us that the transitions are just as important as the poses.

Yoga: Yoga is a state of being, a feeling of union with all that is. It is also a series of practices that include codes of conduct, physical exercises, breathing exercises, and meditation.

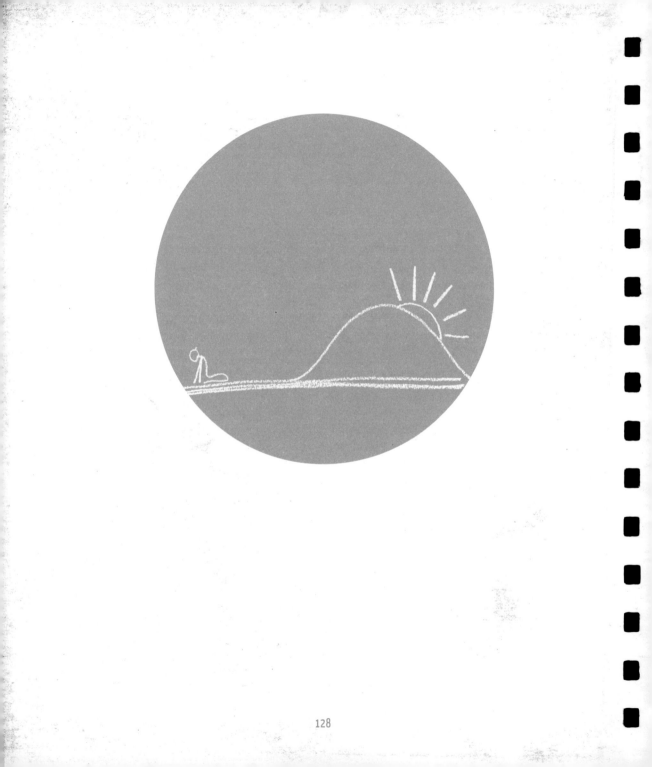